MW01602826

JOE BLOE'S™ GUIDE TO

CHOLESTEROL

JOE BLOE
WITH GARY CHARLES

Published by MSB Books

Montreal, Quebec, Canada MSB — Making Stories Bold

ISBN 978-1-0699039-4-5 (paperback)

ISBN 978-1-0699039-5-2 (ebook)

Cover design by Damonza

Interior design by Laura Boyle

Edited by Dominic Farrell

Printed on demand by Amazon KDP and IngramSpark

Library and Archives Canada Cataloguing in Publication data available upon request.

First Edition

DISCLAIMER

This book is for educational and informational purposes only.

The content in Joe Bloe's Guide to Cholesterol is not intended to diagnose, treat, cure, or prevent any disease, nor should it be interpreted as medical advice. The author is not acting as your physician or healthcare provider.

Health decisions are personal and complex. Always consult a qualified healthcare professional regarding any medical condition, diagnosis, treatment, or change to your diet, medications, or lifestyle.

While every effort has been made to ensure accuracy, medical science evolves, and individual responses vary. The author and publisher assume no responsibility for how the information in this book is used.

This book is meant to help you understand the system — not blindly follow it.

Use your judgment. Ask questions. And when in doubt, seek professional guidance.

For my dad.
If only we knew then what we know now
— about our bodies, our hearts, and the
truth behind the numbers.
This book is both a tribute and a promise:
your lessons were not lost.

CONTENTS

Author's Note

I'm not a physician, cardiologist, or credentialed medical authority. I'm someone who has spent years reading the research most people never see, asking questions most patients never feel empowered to ask, and trying to reconcile a cholesterol conversation that no longer matches the evidence.

This guide is written for everyday readers. It is not meant to replace medical care, diagnose disease, or prescribe treatment. Its purpose is to promote understanding — to explain cholesterol, plaque, and cardiovascular risk in plain language, using the best science available. Everything in this book is grounded in established, peer-reviewed research, including population studies, metabolic trials, imaging data, lipid-particle analysis, and decades of cardiovascular physiology.

For readers who wish to explore further, the sources that informed this guide are listed in the Appendix at the back of the book; a glossary of the scientific terms and concepts used throughout follows the Appendix.

This is not an anti-doctor or anti-medicine book. It is not anti-statin, anti-guideline, or anti-science. Medications have an important place, and clinicians do essential work. But numbers without biological context do not tell the whole story. Modern cardiovascular disease is driven by such things as metabolic dysfunction, inflammation, and environment far more than it is by those things measured in a lab — but public understanding of that has lagged behind that reality.

My goal is simple: to give readers a clearer framework for understanding cholesterol and heart disease, one that reflects where the science has evolved rather than where it once stood. If this guide helps you ask better questions, understand your lab results more clearly, or feel less anxious about a number on a report, then it has done its job.

This book offers no shortcuts and no miracle cures. It offers perspective. And in a healthcare system increasingly built around speed, algorithms, and checklists, perspective may be the most valuable thing patients can get back.

Introduction

I never planned to write a book about cholesterol. For most of my life, my cholesterol level was just another line on my annual blood test. My doctor would point to my LDL (low-density lipoprotein) level, call it "borderline," and I'd nod without really understanding what that meant.

I felt healthy. I had been eating low-carb for years and had kept my weight down. My energy level was good and my blood sugar steady. Yet every appointment ended the same way: "Your LDL is still borderline, and you have borderline hypertension — both risk factors for heart disease."

Borderline became my nickname.

Then came the family-history warning. My father developed angina late in life, and that alone added points to my "risk." It was as if his lifestyle — smoking, stress, poor diet — had somehow fused itself into my DNA. I remember thinking, *So my dad's habits are now my medical destiny?*

My own blood pressure was labeled "essential"

— doctor-speak for *We don't really know why, and we're not digging further.* To me, it wasn't a diagnosis. It was a shrug.

The turning point came during a routine check-up. My doctor opened the Framingham risk calculator, typed in my numbers, and the screen produced a percentage: my "10-year cardiovascular risk." Even though the calculator didn't actually require my LDL, the entire interpretation still revolved around it. In modern cardiology, LDL is the sun, and every other risk factor simply orbits around it. If something in your checkup ends in "DL," you're already halfway to a statin prescription.

He turned the laptop toward me and said, "See? You're at moderate risk. You should start statins."

That was the entire conversation. No discussion of insulin, triglycerides, diet, sleep, stress, inflammation, or overall metabolic health. Just a number generated by an algorithm designed decades ago.

I left the office wondering how a seemingly healthy person — with improving metabolic markers — ends up on the statin conveyor belt.

Later, I emailed my doctor a new study showing that statins offer little or no life-extension benefit for people without existing heart disease. His response wasn't engagement; it was dismissal — not based on reading the paper, but on doubting the abstract. That told me everything. The guideline mattered. The evidence, less so.

Other exchanges reinforced the pattern. When I asked whether lifestyle changes could address blood pressure, I was told hypertension "mostly isn't lifestyle — it's just part of aging." When I requested a homocysteine test, I was asked, "For what reason would you want to do this?"

It became clear I wasn't being evaluated as a person, but as an element in a formula. I was in a system with preloaded conclusions: LDL is the villain, statins are the solution, family history seals the fate.

My doctor wasn't the problem. He's smart and well-intentioned. But he's operating inside a framework that has barely changed in fifty years — one shaped by outdated assumptions, guideline inertia, and risk calculators built before we understood metabolic disease.

My experience with him is what finally pushed me to write this book: he believed I was taking a risk in not starting statins. I believed I would be taking a risk if I blindly followed an outdated model.

Two definitions of risk. Only one reflected modern science.

So I went looking for answers. What I found wasn't a conspiracy — it was a mismatch. A modern environment that has changed faster than our biology is able to adapt, and a medical narrative too narrow to explain what actually causes heart disease.

The truth is, cholesterol isn't the cause of cardiovascular disease; it's a response to deeper problems. Something irritates and inflames the artery wall, oxidizes LDL, and sets the stage for plaque. That "something" isn't cholesterol itself — it's the modern metabolic environment colliding with an ancient physiology.

I've written this book for one simple reason: not to defend cholesterol, not to attack it, but to explain it honestly — without outdated assumptions or pharmaceutical storytelling. You don't need a Ph.D. to understand your own body. You just need someone willing to explain it clearly.

Let's begin.

CHAPTER 1

The Life Molecule

I've read the studies, the transcripts of lectures and expert panels — and not once have I heard a doctor, scientist, or health authority get the basic terminology right. Before we can fix the cholesterol debate, we have to fix the vocabulary.

A molecule is just atoms arranged in a specific way.

Water is H_2O — two hydrogen atoms, one oxygen. Carbon dioxide is CO_2 — one carbon atom, two oxygens.

Simple. Precise. Universal.

Cholesterol is no different. It is one molecule — exactly one — with the chemical formula $C_{27}H_{46}O$: 27 carbon atoms, 46 hydrogen atoms, and a single oxygen. Change even one atom and it is no longer cholesterol.

Chemistry is that precise.

Here's the part nobody ever explains: a cholesterol molecule in your bloodstream is identical to the cholesterol molecule in an egg ... and identical to the one found in fossilized dinosaurs. Same atoms. Same structure. Same molecule.

So where did the concept of "good cholesterol" and "bad cholesterol" come from?

From the same mistake people make when talking about "clean water" and "dirty water."

The water molecule — H_2O — never changes. What changes is the environment. A mountain spring looks "clean," a swamp looks "dirty," but the molecule is the same.

Cholesterol works the same way. There is no good molecule or bad molecule. The environment determines whether cholesterol behaves normally or becomes associated with disease. And this matters, because cholesterol isn't optional — it's essential for life.

The Cholesterol Factory

Your liver is the master builder — the cholesterol factory — and it runs nonstop.

Every day, it manufactures roughly 1,000–1,200 mg of cholesterol. Not because something is wrong, but because cholesterol is far too important to leave to chance.

Your body uses cholesterol everywhere:

- Cell membranes depend on it for structure and flexibility.
- Hormones — estrogen, testosterone, cortisol, progesterone — are built with it.
- The immune system uses it for repair.
- Digestion uses it to create bile acids.
- The nervous system uses enormous amounts to insulate nerves.

Your brain makes up only 2 percent of your body weight but contains almost 20 percent of your cholesterol. Evolution protects this molecule for a reason.

And here's a fact that should have ended the dietary cholesterol panic decades ago:

- Eat more cholesterol → the liver makes less.
- Eat less cholesterol → the liver makes more.

Your body maintains a stable supply because survival depends on it.

So cholesterol was never the villain. The misunderstanding came from confusing the molecule itself with the system that carries it.

A First Look at the Transport System

Before we go further, we need to correct a foundational mistake: LDL and HDL (high-density lipoproteins) are not cholesterol.

They are lipoproteins — transport particles your body uses to move cholesterol and other fats wherever they're needed.

For now, all you need to know is simple: LDL delivers materials outward. HDL returns materials inward.

That's it — they are part of a loop.

Not "good" or "bad."

Not different types of cholesterol.

Just vehicles … part of a system your body relies on every second of your life.

We'll break this system down properly in the next chapter — what these particles are made of, why your liver manufactures them, and how they became so deeply misunderstood.

To Sum Up:

- Cholesterol is one molecule.
- The liver produces most of it.
- Dietary cholesterol barely affects blood levels.
- LDL and HDL are carriers, not cholesterol.
- The molecule is essential for life.

Where Do We Go Next?

In Chapter 2, we meet the particle that became the center of decades of confusion: LDL — the courier blamed for a crime it didn't commit.

This is where the real story begins.

LDL: The "Bad Cholesterol" That Isn't Even Cholesterol

If there's one character in the cholesterol story that has been miscast more than any other, it's LDL. You can walk into almost any doctor's office and still hear the familiar script:

"Your LDL is too high."

"That's your bad cholesterol."

"We need to get that number down."

The term bad cholesterol appears everywhere: in pamphlets, guidelines, drug commercials, TikTok explainers, even medical-school lectures. The mantra LDL is bad cholesterol has been repeated so often that it feels like an unshakable fact.

But the story isn't that simple.

LDL isn't cholesterol.

LDL isn't a molecule.

LDL isn't inherently harmful.

LDL is a transport particle — a courier — produced by the liver to carry vital materials the body depends on for survival.

If LDL vanished tomorrow, the body wouldn't celebrate — it would collapse. Hormone levels would plummet, cell membranes would fall apart, bile acids wouldn't form, nerves would lose their insulation, tissues couldn't repair themselves, and even basic fuel distribution would break down.

LDL isn't the villain. To understand how it ended up with that label, we need to understand what it actually is.

What Is LDL?

LDL stands for low-density lipoprotein — a particle made of fat and protein that transports cholesterol and other essential cargo through the bloodstream. Your liver assembles these particles, loads them with building materials, and sends them out to the tissues that need them.

Each LDL particle has two major components:

The Shell: A flexible coating of phospholipids, proteins, and free cholesterol. This makes the particle water-soluble so it can travel through blood.

The Core: It is made up of cholesteryl esters, triglycerides, and fat-soluble vitamins A, D, E, and K — the raw materials for building and repair cells in the body.

Attached to the surface of each LDL particle is one ApoB (apolipoprotein B-100) molecule — a structural protein that allows the particle to function and serves as its biological "barcode." Without ApoB, LDL particles couldn't circulate or deliver their cargo.

Count the number of ApoB molecules in a sample and you've effectively counted all LDL and related particles. Because every LDL, VLDL (very low-density lipoprotein), IDL (intermediate-density lipoprotein), and Lp(a) (lipoprotein (a)) particle carries one and only one ApoB molecule, the measurement tells you how many particles are in circulation, not just how much cholesterol they're carrying.

What the measurement of the number of ApoB doesn't tell you is size of lipoproteins they're attached to. LDL particles vary in size, and those variations matter. We'll unpack this in the next chapter.

For now, it's enough to understand this: LDL is a courier that transports material necessary for survival. The problems that are associated with it have nothing to do with its design — and everything to do with the environment it travels through.

A Brief Word About HDL

LDL can't be understood without its partner, HDL (high-density lipoprotein). HDL is the return courier. It picks up excess cholesterol from tissues and brings it back to the liver for reuse or repackaging. It's called "high-density" because it carries less fat and more protein, making it smaller and more compact.

LDL delivers.

HDL retrieves.

That's the traffic system — nothing "good" or "bad" about it.

Why This Transport System Exists

Once you realize LDL and HDL are vehicles, the next question becomes obvious: Why do we need vehicles at all?

Because chemistry gives us no choice.

Cholesterol and fat don't dissolve in water — and blood is made up almost entirely of water. Without a carrier, cholesterol would never reach the tissues that depend on it.

Pour olive oil into water and it separates immediately. Cholesterol behaves the same way. The body needed a transport system, so it built one.

In a healthy metabolic environment, this system runs silently and flawlessly. Problems arise only when the environment becomes hostile.

Where the Confusion Began

If LDL is essential for life, and HDL is simply the return trip, how did these particles become labeled "bad" and "good"?

Because early researchers saw the wrong part of the story.

When they opened clogged arteries, they found cholesterol debris, oxidized fats, and damaged LDL particles. What they didn't yet understand were the forces that created the injury: inflammation, oxidative stress, insulin resistance, high blood pressure, mechanical irritation, and seed-oil-driven lipid oxidation.

They saw LDL at the crime scene and assumed it was the criminal.

LDL became "bad."

HDL became "good."

Cholesterol — the molecule itself — was turned into a public enemy.

But here's the truth the last 50 years of research now makes impossible to ignore:

- Cholesterol does not initiate arterial damage.
- LDL shows up because repair has been triggered.

- The environment determines whether LDL completes its job or becomes trapped.

Blaming LDL for heart disease is like blaming ambulances for car crashes because they're always at the scene.

Why LDL Levels Rise — The Explanation Most Doctors Never Offer

Once you see LDL as a courier, the next question becomes obvious: Why do LDL levels go up? And why do levels rise in some of the healthiest people alive?

Because LDL responds to demand — sometimes healthy, sometimes unhealthy.

LDL rises for healthy, adaptive reasons:

- When fasting, LDL helps distribute mobilized fat for fuel.
- During weight loss, stored fat releases and LDL helps move it.
- On low-carb or ketogenic diets, LDL transports more fat because fat becomes your primary fuel.
- During tissue repair or intense training, the body requests more cholesterol to rebuild.
- In pregnancy, LDL rises because a developing baby needs enormous amounts of cholesterol.

None of this is pathology. It's physiology.

LDL also rises in times of metabolic dysfunction: When a person experiences insulin resistance, chronic inflammation, oxidative stress, high triglycerides, or poor sleep, LDL production, clearance, or both become disrupted.

High LDL levels might be the result of normal body operation. Or they might indicate a problem.

Same number. Very different biology.

Yet both people often hear the same prescription: "You need a statin."

This happens when a number becomes a diagnosis.

Why LDL Shows Up in Plaque — the Part Everyone Gets Wrong

If LDL doesn't cause the initial injury, why is it inside plaque?

Because plaque is not a cholesterol spill. Plaque is a chronic wound that never healed.

Arteries can be injured by many stresses — high blood sugar, high insulin, high blood pressure, smoking, seed-oil-driven oxidation, chronic inflammation, visceral fat, or persistent triglyceride overload. The moment the arterial lining is injured, the body launches a repair project — just like it would for a cut on your skin.

Repair requires the exact materials LDL delivers: cholesterol, triglycerides, antioxidants, vitamins.

In a healthy environment, the repair is completed and tissue heals.

In a toxic environment, the repair site never does.

More LDL arrives.

More immune cells arrive.

LDL becomes oxidized.

ApoB becomes distorted.

Macrophages fill with damaged debris, die, and leave behind foam cells — the true core of plaque.

LDL didn't start the injury.

LDL didn't oxidize itself.

LDL didn't "attack" the artery.

The environment damaged LDL.

The immune system attempted repair.

Early researchers mistook presence for cause.

To Sum Up:

- LDL is a courier, not a criminal.
- HDL is its partner, not its opposite.
- The liver drives the system.
- Risk comes from the metabolic environment, not from LDL alone.
- Plaque forms as a result of chronic injury and oxidation — not because cholesterol is drifting through your arteries.

Where Do We Go Next?

It's time to dive into a detail almost no patient is ever told — and yet it changes everything: particle size and particle count.

Why these features matter.

Why they separate harmless LDL from harmful LDL.

And why they explain the contradictions that confuse so many people.

The mystery starts unraveling now.

CHAPTER 3

Size Does Matter

Size matters — at least when it comes to LDL particles. And once you understand why, the whole cholesterol story starts to make far more sense. Large, buoyant LDL particles behave one way; small, dense LDL particles behave another. Size — rarely highlighted on a standard blood test — changes how LDL moves through the bloodstream, how long it lingers, and how it interacts with the arterial wall.

Most people imagine LDL as a single, uniform blob drifting around causing trouble. But LDL isn't one thing. The particles come in different sizes and densities, and those physical traits determine how each behaves. Appreciating this difference is the first step toward understanding your real cardiovascular risk.

Big vs. Small LDL — Two Patterns, Two Behaviors

There are two LDL patterns. The first, Pattern A, is characterized by the prevalence of large, buoyant particles — think beach balls drifting through the bloodstream. Pattern B is characterized by higher levels of smaller, denser particles — more like compact marbles. Both carry cholesterol. Both deliver fat-soluble vitamins, triglycerides, and antioxidants. Both do the same essential job.

But they behave differently because they are built differently. And most importantly, LDL size isn't predetermined by genetics. It adapts to the metabolic environment you create.

Where LDL Comes From — And Why Size Changes

LDL doesn't start out as LDL. Every particle begins life as VLDL — a large, triglyceride-rich "delivery truck" produced by the liver to distribute energy. As VLDL unloads its triglyceride cargo, it shrinks, becoming IDL. This shrinks further and eventually becomes LDL.

This shrinking is normal.

What determines whether LDL stays large and buoyant or shrinks into the small, dense variety is your metabolic state.

LDL size is essentially a real-time reflection of the environment inside your body.

When insulin levels are healthy, triglycerides are stable, and the liver is processing energy efficiently, LDL tends to remain large. When metabolism is strained — particularly in states of insulin resistance — LDL shifts toward the smaller, denser pattern.

How LDL Shrinks — The Metabolic Red Flags

LDL becomes small and dense when the body's internal environment is under stress. High insulin levels, elevated triglycerides, a fatty liver, unstable blood sugar, and chronic metabolic tension keep LDL particles circulating longer than they should. The longer they stay in circulation, the more cargo-swapping they undergo with other lipoproteins. Each exchange strips triglycerides and compacts the particle.

What started as a buoyant beach ball gradually becomes a dense marble.

This transformation is closely tied to insulin resistance. Long before blood sugar rises, elevated insulin disrupts normal lipoprotein clearance. LDL particles accumulate, shrink, and harden. Small, dense LDL isn't "bad" LDL — it's LDL remodeled by a stressed metabolic environment.

What Keeps LDL Large and Buoyant

On the other side of the spectrum, LDL remains large when metabolism functions smoothly. Low triglycerides, stable glucose, healthy insulin signaling, minimal visceral fat, and an efficient liver all allow LDL to deliver its cargo quickly and clear without excessive remodeling.

Up until now, I've used LDL in a general sense; going forward, I'll be more precise — LDL refers to the particle, while LDL-C refers to the cholesterol inside it. Some metabolically healthy individuals may show a high LDL-C (low-density lipoprotein cholesterol) on a standard blood test. The number is elevated not because they are producing dangerous particles, but because each particle is simply carrying more cholesterol. The LDL is doing exactly what it was designed to do.

Why Size Matters More Than the LDL Number

Here's the crucial point: the LDL-C level — the number most people obsess over — measures only the weight of cholesterol inside the particles. It tells you nothing about size of the particle. And size determines behavior.

Two people can produce the same LDL-C value and live in completely different biological realities.

Picture Person A:

- low triglycerides
- high HDL
- stable insulin
- calm inflammation
- a healthy liver

Their LDL is mostly large and buoyant.

Now picture Person B:

- rising triglycerides
- falling HDL
- elevated insulin
- creeping inflammation
- fatty liver
- accumulating visceral fat

Their LDL tends toward the small and dense form.

Same number on a lab report.

Totally different metabolic stories.

Measuring LDL-C alone hides all of this. Without knowing whether the particles are large or small, you're guessing.

LDL Size as a Metabolic Report Card

LDL size quietly reveals the quality of the environment the particles are swimming through. The prevalence of large, buoyant LDL particles generally reflects efficient energy handling, low insulin, stable triglycerides, and a calm liver. Elevated levels of small, dense LDL particles often signal insulin resistance, lipid congestion, high triglycerides, and chronic metabolic strain.

And here's an important distinction: you don't need to be overweight to make small LDL. Pattern B LDL can be found in thin people with high insulin or hidden visceral fat. Likewise, you don't have to be ultra lean to make large LDL. These particles aren't responding to your waistline — they're responding to your chemistry.

Where We Go Next

Now you understand LDL's "two personalities": big and buoyant versus small and dense. But neither type — on its own — is the real danger. The real issue is what happens next: plaque formation.

What Exactly Is Plaque?

Before we interpret lab results, we need to answer the most fundamental question in the field: What exactly is plaque?

Not the cartoon version of it. Not "cholesterol sludge." The real biological structure.

It's time to talk about what it's made of, what triggers its formation, why some plaques remain quiet for decades, and why others rupture without warning.

Most people can't explain what it is.

Many doctors describe it incompletely.

Once you truly understand what plaque is, everything else — the role of LDL, statins, diet, metabolic health — finally makes sense.

It's time to meet the real villain.

CHAPTER 4

The Enemy Isn't LDL — It's Plaque

If you ask the average person what plaque is, they'll say something like, "That's the cholesterol that clogs your arteries." It's the image we've all been fed: cholesterol piling up like gunk in a pipe until one day the whole thing shuts down.

It's simple.

It's visual.

And it's wrong.

Plaque isn't cholesterol any more than a house fire is made of firefighters. Yes, plaque contains cholesterol — much of it delivered by LDL — but cholesterol didn't start the fire, and it doesn't explain why it keeps burning. Plaque is something else entirely: a messy, chaotic biological construction site that never got cleaned up.

If you want to understand heart attacks and strokes, you need to understand what plaque actually is. Once you grasp its true nature, the entire story of cardiovascular disease changes.

What Plaque Really Is — and What It Isn't

The biggest myth is that plaque is cholesterol stuck to the artery wall like sludge. That's cartoon biology. Plaque is made of inflamed tissue, dead immune cells, oxidized lipids, connective fibers, and sometimes calcium—not sludge, but a failed repair job, a wound that never healed. All of this sits inside the arterial wall, not in the artery like debris in a pipe.

Imagine a road crew trying to fix the same pothole day after day, but traffic never stops long enough for the job to be finished. The repair becomes permanent chaos.

That chaos is plaque.

LDL didn't cause the pothole — it brought repair materials. But because the wound never closed, those materials mix with oxidized fats and dead immune cells. This is where LDL size becomes relevant: large, buoyant LDL tends to deliver its cargo and leave, while small, dense LDL can slip more easily into an irritated arterial wall and linger in that unstable environment. The longer it lingers, the more likely it is to become oxidized and trapped. Particle size doesn't make LDL "good" or "bad" — it changes how LDL behaves at a repair site.

That mixture — inflamed tissue, dead immune cells, oxidized lipids, connective fibers, and sometimes calcium — is plaque.

What Plaque Actually Looks Like

Under a microscope, plaque doesn't resemble hardened cholesterol at all. Soft plaque — the dangerous kind — looks like wet drywall: unstable, inflamed, crowded with dead macrophages and oxidized fats. Hard plaque is different. Over time, the body tries to stabilize the chaos by laying down calcium, creating a tougher, more rigid structure. It's not ideal, but it's far less likely to rupture.

Soft plaque is the villain.

Hard plaque is the scar.

One is explosive; the other is old damage.

How Plaque Begins

It always starts with something tiny: a microscopic scrape or irritated patch on the endothelium, the inner lining of an artery. You never feel the damage — there are no nerves there. Your body reacts instantly. LDL arrives carrying cholesterol for new membranes, triglycerides for energy, and fat-soluble antioxidants. Immune cells gather to coordinate repair. In a healthy metabolic environment, the wound closes and the artery returns to normal.

But if the irritation keeps happening — repeated glucose spikes, chronically high insulin, oxidative stress, hypertension, inflammatory chemicals released by visceral fat — the site never fully heals. LDL keeps arriving. Immune cells keep arriving. The construction zone stays open permanently. Over time, debris builds up. Eventually the repair site isn't a repair site anymore. It's a fixture.

That fixture is plaque.

Why Soft Plaque Is the Killer

The body hates instability. When a wound refuses to heal, it tries to contain the chaos by laying down calcium — creating calcified plaque. That plaque is older, more rigid, and far less likely to rupture.

Soft plaque, however, is inflamed and fragile, protected by only a thin fibrous cap. One surge in blood pressure or inflammation can tear that cap. When it ruptures, the body panics and sends a clot to seal the injury. Inside a coronary artery, that clot can block blood flow in seconds and trigger a heart attack. Inside an artery feeding the brain, the same mechanism produces a stroke.

Different organs, same biology.

Plaque causes harm not by slowly clogging an artery, but by rupturing and triggering a clot — a mechanism we'll explore in more detail shortly.

And because there are no symptoms associated with the buildup of soft plaque, most people never see it coming.

Calcification: What It Means — and Doesn't

When plaque hardens, forget the idea that cholesterol is "turning to stone." Calcification is the body's attempt to stabilize a wound that never healed. A high coronary artery calcium (CAC) score indicates that you have older, calcified plaque. A score of zero means there is no detectable calcified plaque — but it tells you nothing about soft plaque. Soft plaque appears first and can exist long before calcium shows up. This is why someone with a CAC of zero can still have a cardiovascular event.

Calcification is the scar.

Soft plaque is the wound.

Why Plaque Grows Silently

The buildup of plaque gives no warning signs. Arteries don't have pain receptors on the inside. They can be irritated for years without you feeling a thing. That's why the first symptom is often the event — a heart attack or stroke. It isn't sudden. It's silent.

The Environment That Feeds Plaque

Plaque doesn't form randomly. It grows in an unhealthy metabolic environment — the exact environment modern life creates perfectly. High-fasting insulin, repeated glucose spikes, oxidative stress, elevated triglycerides, fatty liver, inflammation driven by visceral fat, poor sleep, chronic stress, seed-oil-heavy diets, smoking, and hypertension all contribute to an atmosphere where arterial injuries never fully heal.

LDL becomes dangerous only in this environment.

Same particle.

Different environments.

Different outcomes.

Why LDL Gets Blamed

Early researchers saw LDL fragments inside plaque and assumed LDL caused the disease. It was a simple idea to teach and easy to market. But LDL is present for a different reason: it brings necessary molecules to help heal an injury. The problem wasn't the particle — it was the environment that damaged it and trapped it there. Once that misunderstanding took hold, however, LDL became the villain in a story that was never biologically accurate.

Why Lowering LDL Isn't Enough

Lowering LDL reduces the number of delivery trucks. But it doesn't fix the pothole. If inflammation and metabolic stress remain, the wound stays open. People with low LDL can still have heart attacks. People with high LDL but excellent metabolic health often don't. LDL is not the central variable. The environment is.

What Stabilizes — and Sometimes Reverses — the Buildup of Plaque

Here's the encouraging part: plaque is not destiny. When the metabolic environment calms down, soft plaque stabilizes and often shrinks. Lower inflammation, improved insulin sensitivity, reduced visceral fat, normalized triglycerides, steady liver function, lower blood pressure, and reduced arterial irritation all help stabilize the wound. As the chaos resolves, soft plaque frequently develops a thicker, more protective cap — a fragile spot becomes something far safer.

Hard plaque may remain, but the dangerous kind — soft, unstable plaque — shrinks when the storm ends. The body wants to heal. It just needs the chaos to stop.

Sidebar: "Hardening of the Arteries" — A Misleading Phrase

You've probably heard atherosclerosis described as "hardening of the arteries." That phrase has stuck — but it points in the wrong direction.

Arteries don't harden because cholesterol slowly builds up like mineral scale in a pipe. The hardening comes later, after years of injury and failed repair inside the arterial wall, when the body responds by laying down calcium to stabilize soft, unstable plaque — a process known as calcification.

In other words, "hardening" describes how arteries can look at the end of the process — not what caused the disease in the first place.

If you focus only on hardening, you miss the real problem: ongoing damage that never fully heals.

The Real Villain: Unstable Plaque

Strip away the slogans and oversimplified messaging, and the picture becomes clear: LDL isn't the problem. Soft, unstable plaque is. And that kind of plaque forms only in a damaged metabolic environment, one marked by inflammation, oxidative stress, insulin resistance, and constant arterial irritation.

When you improve that environment, you don't just "lower risk," you change the biology that makes plaque dangerous in the first place.

Now that you know plaque is a failed repair — not a pile of cholesterol — the next question becomes inevitable: If plaque is the real threat … why aren't we measuring it?

CHAPTER 5

If Plaque Is the Problem, Why Aren't We Measuring Plaque?

Before we go any further, it's worth recapping.

- Cholesterol is a molecule. A real molecule with a fixed formula: $C_{27}H_{46}O$. That formula never changes.
- There is no "good" or "bad" cholesterol; those labels describe types of lipoproteins, not cholesterol itself. Cholesterol is cholesterol, the same molecule animals have used for millions of years.
- Your liver makes cholesterol — intentionally — because every cell in your body requires it for structure, repair, hormones, and survival.
- LDL provides transportation. It's the delivery vehicle that carries cholesterol from the liver

to the rest of the body. It is not the cargo; it's the truck.

- And here's the crucial point: the truck isn't the danger. Plaque is. Specifically, soft, unstable plaque forming inside the arterial wall. Atherosclerosis isn't cholesterol sticking to a pipe. It's a wound that never fully heals.

Put all that together and an obvious question emerges:

If plaque is the real problem … why aren't we measuring plaque?

It should be straightforward. Plaque drives heart attacks. Plaque drives strokes. Plaque determines risk. Yet despite this, plaque is rarely assessed directly.

Modern cardiology often operates with a kind of blindfold on. Physicians focus on LDL numbers, use population formulas to estimate disease, and make major treatment decisions without confirming whether a patient has plaque at all. It's like treating a fever without taking a temperature, or guessing whether your car needs gas without checking the gauge, or trying to fix a leak without ever seeing the pipe.

In every other field of medicine, the rule is simple: measure the thing you're trying to treat. But in heart disease — the leading cause of death in the modern world — we measure LDL, the delivery truck, instead of plaque, the hazard.

Doctors aren't negligent. They're following guidelines rooted in an era when LDL was easy to measure and plaque was not. Those guidelines stuck, even as technology changed. So we continue estimating plaque instead of imaging it.

But estimation isn't measurement. It's guesswork dressed up as precision.

The contradiction becomes obvious once you see it: We define the disease by plaque, prove outcomes by plaque, warn patients about plaque — and then make decisions without actually checking for plaque.

Millions of people are placed on lifelong medication without ever learning whether they have plaque at all. Once you recognize how backwards that is, the blindfold becomes impossible to ignore.

The Tools Already Exist — We Just Don't Use Them

There are ways to measure plaque. The **Coronary Artery Calcium (CAC) Scan**, for example, is a low-dose CT scan that detects calcified plaque in the coronary arteries. No needles, no treadmill, no dye. You lie down, hold your breath, and you're done.

A CAC score provides something a standard cholesterol test never will: direct evidence of disease.

Not a probability.

Not an estimate.

Actual plaque.

A CAC of zero typically means there is no detectable calcified plaque and very low short-term risk — even if LDL is high. A higher score means there is calcified plaque, i.e., plaque that has been forming for years.

So, CAC tells a story: a score above zero means stabilization has begun, which means atherosclerosis has existed for years. But CAC scans have their limitations: they cannot see early soft plaque. A zero score means no calcified plaque — not necessarily "no plaque at all."

Despite its value, CAC remains underused, partly because it is often paid out of pocket.

A **Carotid Intima-Media Thickness (CIMT)** test uses ultrasound to measure the thickness of the artery wall in the neck and can reveal early, soft plaque long before calcification appears. It is one of the most useful, non-invasive tools for measuring early atherosclerotic changes.

Coronary Computed Tomography Angiography (CCTA) goes even further, visualizing both calcified and soft plaque. It's extraordinarily informative, but it requires contrast dye and exposes patients to radiation, so it isn't used for routine screening.

The **Ankle–Brachial Index (ABI)** compares blood pressure at the arm and ankle to assess blood flow. It doesn't show plaque directly, but a low ABI strongly suggests systemic atherosclerosis. Like other screening tools, it offers a clue — not a diagnosis — that cholesterol numbers often miss.

The point is simple:
We can see plaque.
We can measure plaque.
We can track plaque.
Some tools detect calcified plaque.
Some detect soft plaque.
Some detect both.
Yet most people never hear about these tests.
Most doctors never mention them.
And millions continue receiving treatment for a disease they've never been scanned for.
This is the irony of modern cardiology: We finally have windows into the arteries —
but we're still managing patients with the blinds pulled shut.

CHAPTER 6

If Plaque Is the Enemy, What Can Be Done?

If you've followed the story so far, you already see the core truth modern cardiology keeps missing: plaque — not LDL — is the real threat. And plaque doesn't appear out of nowhere. It is the product of a damaged metabolic environment, the biological equivalent of a construction site that never closes.

So the natural question is: If plaque is what kills, what can we actually do about it?

Here's the first surprise most people never hear in a doctor's office: no medication melts plaque. Not statins, not PCSK9 inhibitors, not niacin, ezetimibe, or GLP-1 agonists. The Hollywood fantasy of arteries "clogged with gunk" that can be flushed out by a solvent is just that: a fantasy. But it isn't how biology works.

But that doesn't mean the drugs are useless. Far from it.

Modern cardiology excels at stabilizing plaque. When plaque stabilizes, the fibrous cap thickens, inflammation cools, and the lesion becomes far less likely to rupture. And rupture — not narrowing — is what triggers heart attacks and strokes.

Statins don't melt plaque, but they reduce inflammation within the lesion and may slightly shrink the soft core. PCSK9 inhibitors dramatically lower LDL and quiet the biological turbulence inside unstable plaques. These drugs don't "clean" arteries; they make dangerous plaques behave more like scars than grenades. This is why cardiologists rely on them, especially after an event.

But even the best medications can't overcome a toxic metabolic environment. If insulin remains high, glucose unstable, triglycerides elevated, liver fat accumulating, inflammation rising, or seed oils driving oxidative stress, plaque continues forming in the background.

You can't stabilize a burning building by repainting the walls.

And this leads to the truth that prevention-focused physicians understand: plaque regression happens only when the metabolic environment improves. Imaging studies repeatedly show that when insulin drops, triglycerides fall, endothelial function improves, nitric oxide rises, liver fat shrinks, and inflammatory signaling cools, the body finally gets the chance to close the wound. Soft plaque stabilizes — and in some cases, slowly shrinks.

Millimeter by millimeter, the biology changes.

If the environment doesn't improve, LDL — high or low — will continue to reflect the chaos. That's why people with "normal" LDL still have heart attacks, and why metabolically healthy people with high LDL often don't. LDL was never the master switch. The environment was.

That's why functional-medicine physicians and prevention-oriented cardiologists ask a different set of questions. They don't begin with "How do we suppress LDL?" They begin by asking:

What's inflaming this artery?

Why is LDL oxidizing here?

What is irritating the endothelium?

What's happening in the liver, fat tissue, or bloodstream that's turning a repair molecule into a hazard?

They follow the biology upstream instead of medicating the biomarkers downstream.

So what can be done about plaque?

A great deal — but none of it starts with a pill.

Insulin is the first lever. Chronically high insulin irritates the endothelium and fuels arterial inflammation. Lowering insulin — by reducing sugars, refined carbohydrates, alcohol, and constant snacking — gives the artery lining a chance to reset.

Triglycerides are the next piece in the puzzle. Elevated triglycerides signal impaired fat metabolism and correlate strongly with soft plaque. Remove sugars, alcohol, ultra-processed foods, and especially industrial seed oils, and triglycerides often fall rapidly.

Inflammation is the accelerant. It keeps plaque soft, unstable, and fragile. Better sleep, lower stress, greater sunlight exposure, steady low-intensity movement, and reductions in visceral fat all help cool the inflamed environment.

Then comes endothelial function. Healthy endothelium cells produce nitric oxide, a molecule that keeps arteries flexible and resilient. When nitric oxide rises, plaque formation slows. Pomegranate, beets, leafy greens, sunlight, nasal breathing, and zone-2 cardio all support this natural anti-atherosclerotic system.

And that brings us to the most commonly overlooked disruptor: industrial seed oils.

These omega-6-rich oils — canola, soybean, corn, cottonseed, sunflower, safflower, grapeseed — dominate modern food production. They are cheap and shelf-stable, but they are extremely prone to oxidation. They distort cell membranes, impair mitochondrial function, and fuel the oxidative stress that makes LDL dangerous in the first place. These oils accumulate in fat tissue for years, altering the metabolic environment in ways most people never consider.

Remove them, and everything changes. LDL oxidizes less. Triglycerides fall. Liver fat improves. Visceral fat recedes. Arteries relax. The entire system quiets.

This isn't fringe.

It's biochemistry.

Exercise supports this environment further. Zone-2 cardio strengthens mitochondria. Strength training reduces visceral fat. Walking enhances endothelial health. It doesn't require marathons — only consistency.

Even breathing matters. High stress elevates cortisol; cortisol raises blood pressure; and high pressure increases rupture risk. Slow nasal breathing and longer exhalations measurably improve arterial tone. Small choices accumulate.

So what can actually be done about plaque?

Make changes to the environment that created it.

Plaque becomes dangerous only when the environment is dangerous. Fix the environment — lower insulin, calm inflammation, restore nitric oxide, eliminate seed oils, improve sleep, move your body — and plaque stops behaving like a grenade. It stabilizes, quiets, and in many people, slowly regresses.

It cannot be rushed.

It cannot be hacked.

But it can absolutely be done.

The real battle isn't inside the artery wall.

It's in the world the artery lives in.

Change that world, and plaque becomes manageable. Ignore it, and no medication in the world can protect you from a metabolic fire.

CHAPTER 7

What Really Happens During a Heart Attack or Stroke?

We've seen that plaque — specifically the soft, unstable kind tucked inside the wall of an artery — is the precursor to cardiovascular disease. So the next question is this: How does that plaque actually turn into a heart attack or stroke?

The Quiet Before the Rupture

Dangerous plaque almost never causes symptoms. Arteries don't have pain receptors on the inside, so irritation and inflammation remain completely silent. You can have modest arterial narrowing for years and feel perfectly normal. Most people have no idea anything is wrong because the trouble doesn't come from the slow buildup — it comes from an abrupt rupture.

The Moment the Fibrous Cap Breaks

Soft plaque is covered by a thin fibrous "cap," like drywall concealing damp insulation. That cap can stay intact for years — until something creates enough stress to tear it open. A spike in blood pressure, a burst of adrenaline, an inflammatory flare, even the normal bending of an artery during exercise can be enough. You wouldn't feel the tear. But your body does.

The Body Reacts: "We're Bleeding — Seal It Now."

A ruptured plaque looks to the body like internal bleeding. The emergency response is immediate: platelets rush in, clotting factors activate, and fibrin strands weave a mesh to seal the injury. Within seconds, a clot forms on top of the ruptured plaque. The body is trying to save your life, but when this happens in an artery supplying the heart or brain, that same lifesaving reflex can be lethal. The clot doesn't stay small; it grows until it blocks the artery completely.

A Heart Attack: Blood Stops, Muscle Suffocates

If the blockage occurs in a coronary artery — one that supplies the heart — oxygen delivery stops. First the heart muscle struggles, then it suffocates, and then it dies. People imagine heart attacks as slow "clogs," like kitchen grease building up in a pipe. The truth is, they occur far more suddenly: a hidden plaque ruptures, a clot forms, the artery closes, and the heart tissue downstream loses its lifeline. This entire sequence can unfold in minutes, which is why someone can feel fine one day and collapse the next.

A Stroke: Same Mechanism, Different Organ

Ischemic strokes — the most common type — occur in exactly the same way. A plaque ruptures in a vessel feeding the brain, a clot forms, blood flow stops, and brain cells begin dying. Heart attack or stroke — same mechanism. Only the location changes.

Why Some Plaques Kill and Others Stay Quiet

The plaques that rupture are not usually the big ones. A large, calcified plaque may narrow an artery, but it tends to be stable. The small, soft, inflamed plaques — the ones that barely narrow the artery at all — are the ones that rupture easily. This is why people with "normal" stress tests can still have heart attacks, why someone whose imaging shows mild narrowing of the arteries can collapse the next week, and why a zero-calcium score doesn't rule out early soft plaque. The tiniest unstable plaque can be deadly.

Why Most People Never Feel a Warning

One of the cruelest realities is that your first symptom of heart disease may be your heart attack. Plaque buildup is silent. The rupture — not the buildup — creates symptoms. Relying on "how you feel" is one of the most dangerous strategies imaginable.

The Real Story: A Cardiovascular Event Is a Clot, Not a Clog

Strip away the decades of misleading imagery and the pattern appears clearly: a soft plaque ruptures, a clot forms, blood flow stops, and the organ downstream suffocates. That is a heart attack. That is a stroke. The goal isn't to "lower cholesterol." The goal is to stabilize plaque and fix the environment that makes rupture possible in the first place.

Where We Go Next

Now that you understand what a cardiovascular event actually is — and why it happens so suddenly — you're ready for the next chapter: What do all these blood tests really mean? And how do you know which numbers matter?

CHAPTER 8

So, You've Had a Cholesterol Test

Let's start with a simple truth: You've never actually had a "cholesterol test."

What you've had is a lipid panel — a test that measures the carriers that transport cholesterol, not the cholesterol molecule itself. Cholesterol has a fixed chemical identity ($C_{27}H_{46}O$); it doesn't come in "good" or "bad" forms. The lipoproteins do.

Because we still call this a "cholesterol test," most people assume the numbers on the page represent cholesterol directly. They don't. They represent the mass of cholesterol being carried by various particles — LDL, HDL, VLDL — each performing a transport job that keeps you alive.

And the value that usually gets circled — LDL-C — is one of the most misunderstood numbers in medicine.

The LDL-C score doesn't count LDL particles.

It doesn't describe particle size.

It doesn't reveal oxidation, inflammation, or metabolic stress.

It simply measures the amount of cholesterol mass packed inside your LDL particles.

Two people can have the same LDL-C and live in completely different metabolic realities. One may produce large, stable LDL particles inside a healthy metabolic environment. Another may produce small, dense LDL particles shaped by insulin resistance, inflammation, and liver overload.

Same number. Opposite biology.

This is why understanding your lipid panel — truly understanding it — means looking past the headline numbers and into the context that actually predicts cardiovascular health.

Let's break down what each value means, why some have been misused for decades, and why others deserve far more attention.

LDL-C — A Number Whose Target Won't Stop Moving

The value of LDL-C as a marker rose to prominence in the 1970s, not because it is the best indicator of risk, but because it was the easiest to measure. Once guidelines were built around it, LDL-C became the gravitational center of cardiology — even as better science emerged.

What most people never hear is that the LDL-C "cutoffs" have been drifting downward for decades:

In the 1970s and '80s, 160 mg/dL was considered normal.

In the 1990s, the bar dropped to 130.

By the 2000s, "optimal" was defined as under 100.

Today, in certain categories, targets as low as 70 or even 55 are recommended.

The human body hasn't changed.

The targets did.

And as the threshold continues to drop, millions more people become candidates for statins — a topic explored in depth later.

LDL-C still tells you something. But it tells you nothing about

- how many LDL particles you actually have;
- whether they are large or small;
- whether your arteries are inflamed;
- whether plaque exists;
- whether your metabolic environment is stable or collapsing.

The LDL-C test measures cargo, not risk.

Without context, it is an incomplete story.

Non-HDL Cholesterol — A Slightly Smarter Version

Non-HDL cholesterol (total cholesterol minus HDL) includes cholesterol carried by all apoB-containing particles — LDL, VLDL, IDL, and Lp(a). It's a broader measure than LDL-C and performs better in people with high triglycerides.

But it still doesn't count particles or describe their size.

It's a small upgrade from the standard test, but it doesn't give a full answer.

ApoB — Counting the Vehicles, Not the Cargo

Apolipoprotein B (ApoB-100) is the identifying protein found on every atherogenic particle: LDL, VLDL, IDL, and

Lp(a). Each particle carries exactly one ApoB protein.

That means a measure of ApoB isn't an estimate.

It's a count.

And counts matter because plaque isn't formed from loose cholesterol molecules — it forms when particles slip into a damaged arterial wall. More particles mean more opportunities.

Typical clinical interpretations:

- Over 90 mg/dL → High risk
- 80-89 mg/dL → Moderate risk
- Less than 80 mg/dL → Low risk

But even ApoB counts must be interpreted in context. An ApoB of 100 in a metabolically healthy person with low triglycerides and high HDL tells a very different story than the same ApoB count in someone with insulin resistance and chronic inflammation.

Particle count matters.

But the world those particles live in matters more.

HDL — Not "Good Cholesterol," but a Return Vehicle

HDL is not "good cholesterol." It's simply the courier that transports cholesterol back to the liver.

High HDL typically accompanies strong metabolic health.

Low HDL often signals metabolic strain — insulin resistance, liver stress, inflammation, or visceral fat.

HDL becomes even more meaningful when paired with triglycerides.

Triglycerides — The Metabolic Truth Detector

Few numbers on your panel reveal as much as the triglyceride count.

High triglycerides almost always indicate elevated insulin, liver congestion, unstable glucose, or chronic inflammation.

Low triglycerides signal metabolic stability.

A rough guide:

- Under 90 mg/dL — excellent
- 90–150 — borderline
- Over 150 — metabolic stress
- Over 200 — almost always insulin resistance

Triglycerides tell you more about metabolic health than LDL-C ever will.

The TG (triglycerides):HDL Ratio — The Hidden Decoder

This one ratio predicts LDL behavior better than LDL-C:

TG:HDL ratio = triglycerides ÷ HDL

A ratio below ~1.5 suggests a predominance of large, buoyant LDL; above 3.0 strongly indicates insulin resistance and a shift toward small, dense LDL.

This ratio costs nothing to calculate and often reveals more than the doctor's circled LDL number.

LDL Size — The Variable Most Lipid Panels Ignore

LDL comes in different sizes. Large LDL behaves very differently than small LDL.

Small, dense LDL lingers longer, oxidizes easily, and slips into irritated arterial walls. Larger particles are far more benign.

Standard lipid panels don't measure LDL size.

The test that does — NMR Lipoprotein Analysis — is rarely included.

Why?

Take your pick:

- It complicates the LDL-only narrative.
- It doesn't serve drug-first guideline simplicity.
- It forces doctors to talk about metabolism rather than one number.

Let's just say, there is no biological reason for it to be excluded.

NMR measures LDL particle count (LDL-P), LDL size, VLDL patterns, and HDL subfractions. In other words, it finally answers the question LDL-C can't:

What kind of LDL do you actually have?

NMR doesn't diagnose plaque, but it shows when plaque-forming conditions are present.

Lp(a) — The One-Time Test Everyone Should Request

Lp(a) is an LDL-like particle with an additional protein attached that makes plaque stickier and more rupture-prone. Its presence is almost always a genetic feature.

You only need to measure it once in your life.

A high Lp(a) doesn't guarantee disease; it simply means the metabolic environment around it must be impeccable.

Putting It All Together — The Pattern Is the Point

No single number from a lipid panel can predict cardiovascular risk on its own. The story emerges only when you read the pattern.

- LDL-C measures cholesterol mass.
- HDL reflects metabolic resilience.
- Triglyceride levels expose insulin resistance.
- TG:HDL predicts LDL behavior.
- ApoB tests count atherogenic particles.
- Lp(a) reveals inherited risk.
- NMR (when used) identifies dangerous particle patterns.

If triglycerides are low, HDL strong, ApoB reasonable, and the TG:HDL ratio healthy, LDL will usually behave as designed — as a transport vehicle, not a threat.

When the metabolic environment degrades, LDL gets blamed for the damage caused by everything around it.

The real question isn't, Is your LDL high?

The real question is: *What kind of environment is your LDL living in?*

Because LDL is not dangerous by nature.

It becomes dangerous inside a damaged metabolic world.

Now that you understand what your lipid panel is actually measuring — and what it isn't — you're ready for the questions people fear most:

What does it really mean when LDL is high?

And how do you know when it matters — and when it doesn't?

CHAPTER 9

The Great Food Reversal

For decades, the public was told a simple story: saturated fat is deadly, dietary cholesterol is dangerous, and foods like eggs, butter, and red meat are ticking time bombs. The advice sounds authoritative. It came from doctors, dietitians, public-health agencies, cereal companies, margarine manufacturers — anyone with a microphone.

But the advice wasn't just wrong.

It inverted reality.

Before we dive into the modern food chain — seed oils, processed snacks, artificial dyes, engineered sweetness — we need to revisit the foods that were demonized first. The misunderstanding began here, and the fallout still shapes the way people eat today.

Eggs — The Perfect Food That Became a Scapegoat

Eggs contain cholesterol — the same molecule that our bodies produce. That single fact put them on the nutritional blacklist for nearly forty years. People were told to limit eggs, avoid yolks, or replace them with "heart-healthy" substitutes.

Then the science caught up.

The liver produces about one gram of cholesterol per day because every cell requires it. When dietary cholesterol rises, the liver makes less; when dietary cholesterol falls, the liver makes more. The body regulates this with microscopic precision because cholesterol is essential.

Eggs were never the problem.

The guidelines were.

By the mid-2010s, major health agencies quietly admitted that dietary cholesterol is not a nutrient of concern. But the stigma lingered — a perfect example of how slowly bad advice dies.

Butter — Blamed, Replaced, and Then Exonerated

Butter was condemned for the same reasons as eggs: it contains saturated fat and cholesterol. Early researchers assumed saturated fat raised LDL-C, which they believed clogged arteries. Using that logic, butter was deemed the villain and margarine became the savior.

But margarine isn't a harmless substitute. It's made from hydrogenated seed oils — industrial trans fats — chemically altered to be shelf-stable and marketed as "heart-healthy."

It turns out to be anything but.

Trans fats increase inflammation, damage arteries, lower HDL, and raise cardiovascular risk more than butter ever

56

could. The "healthier choice" caused more harm than the food it replaced.

When the evidence became overwhelming, trans fats were banned. Labels changed. Formulas were rewritten. But there was no apology, no reckoning, no explanation for how such a colossal mistake misled the public for half a century.

Butter isn't the failure.

The science that condemned it was.

What never came with that reversal was an apology. There was no moment where doctors, dietitians, pharmaceutical companies, or public health agencies said, "We were wrong about butter and eggs." No acknowledgment of decades of fear, restriction, or misplaced blame. The advice simply changed — quietly — and the institutions that promoted it moved on.

Red Meat — The Myth That Refuses to Die

Eggs recovered. Butter recovered. Margarine collapsed.

But red meat? Still stuck in nutritional purgatory.

The fear came from the same outdated logic: saturated fat raises LDL-C, therefore red meat must cause heart disease. No nuance about LDL particle size. No discussion of inflammation, insulin resistance, triglycerides, metabolic health, nutrient density, or bioavailability.

Even today, many anti-meat studies rely on weak food-frequency questionnaires and tiny statistical associations — usually in populations eating meat alongside fries, buns, soft drinks, and seed-oil-fried everything. Blaming the steak for the fast-food meal is like blaming the piano for the bar fight.

The evidence never matched the fear.

If eggs and butter were wrongly condemned, it's fair to ask why red meat is still presumed guilty.

So What Was the Real Mistake?

Dietary cholesterol was only recently acknowledged as a non-factor in so-called "high cholesterol." And it's worthwhile pausing to consider that fact. The cholesterol we're talking about here is the same molecule we met back in Chapter 1 — plain cholesterol, with a fixed structure. It isn't LDL. It isn't HDL. It isn't a lipoprotein at all.

Which raises an obvious question. If dietary cholesterol — the molecule itself — was never the problem, why does the conversation still revolve around "lowering cholesterol"? Why focus on suppressing a molecule the body carefully regulates rather than the environment that damages arteries in the first place?

Now that we've cleared away the first layer of myths, we can ask the question that frames the next chapter:

How did the war on natural foods begin?

That story starts with one man — and one of the most influential nutrition errors of the 20th century.

CHAPTER 10

Ancel Keys and the Birth of Fat Fear

In October 1955, President Dwight D. Eisenhower collapsed during a mid-afternoon round of golf. The diagnosis — a myocardial infarction — shocked the country. If the President could have a heart attack, anyone could. Overnight, cardiovascular disease became a national obsession.

Almost no one mentioned Eisenhower's decades of smoking — three to four packs a day, stopped only months before the event. Smoking is a major cause of heart disease, but naming tobacco as the villain was politically, economically, and culturally inconvenient. America wanted a simpler explanation, something tied to personal choice and diet.

Americans looking for a diagnosis turned to a confident physiologist from the University of Minnesota: Ancel Keys.

Keys had studied metabolism and starvation, not heart disease. But he offered something irresistible: a clean, digestible formula the public could memorize in one sentence:

Saturated fat → higher cholesterol → heart disease.

It was simple.

It was elegant.

And after Eisenhower's scare, the country was ready to believe it.

The Seven Countries Study — When a Hypothesis Became a Map

To validate his theory, Keys launched the Seven Countries Study, following more than 12,000 men across seven nations. His conclusion looked compelling: populations that ate more saturated fat experienced more heart disease.

The medical world applauded. Textbooks adopted the message. Public-health organizations repeated it with absolute confidence.

But the neat conclusion came with problems.

First, not all available countries were included. Keys initially examined data from 22 nations but selected only the seven that fit his proposed pattern. When all 22 were graphed, the correlation between saturated fat and heart disease faded dramatically.

Second, some of the chosen countries contradicted his message.

Japan ate animal protein and fat yet had low heart disease — largely due to low sugar consumption and minimal processed food. France consumed high amounts of saturated fat but had low heart-disease rates — the "French Paradox," which wasn't a paradox at all, just data that didn't fit the hypothesis.

Third, sugar and refined carbohydrates were barely considered. Keys zoomed in on a single nutrient while ignoring the broader metabolic environment.

Keys wasn't acting with ill intent. But his focus became doctrine — not because it was perfect science, but because it offered a story institutions could use.

Why Keys' Theory Was So Attractive

Looking back, it's easy to wonder how one man's hypothesis reshaped global nutrition policy. But the appeal was obvious.

It was simple. A simple narrative with a single villain is easier to communicate than one with a complex metabolic landscape.

It was measurable. Cholesterol could be tested. Saturated fat could be quantified. Public-health agencies love measurable targets.

It shifted attention away from smoking. The tobacco industry benefited from LDL becoming the scapegoat.

It aligned perfectly with food-industry interests. Companies could reformulate products to be "low-fat," replacing fat with sugar, starch, and industrial oils — cheap ingredients with long shelf lives.

It matched the cultural moment. Post-war America embraced modernity, technology, and scientific authority. If an expert said saturated fat was dangerous, people listened.

The hypothesis wasn't proven — but it was useful. And useful ideas spread much faster than accurate ones.

When Hypothesis Became Law

In 1961, the American Heart Association released the first official guidelines telling Americans to restrict saturated fat. A few years later, Time magazine put Keys on its cover, turning him into the face of heart-disease prevention.

From there, the cascade was unstoppable.

Grocery stores filled with low-fat yogurts, low-fat salad dressings, low-fat cereals, margarine, and processed "diet foods." Fat was removed. Sugar and refined carbs replaced it. Vegetable oils flooded every aisle.

Medical treatments improved — lowering heart-attack mortality — but the population became metabolically sicker. Obesity climbed. Diabetes surged. Fatty liver disease appeared. The very diet meant to prevent heart disease helped trigger a metabolic crisis.

Keys solved a political problem, not a biological one.

The LDL Era — A Simplistic Villain Is Born

Keys didn't just demonize saturated fat, he elevated cholesterol as the central villain in heart disease. As lipoprotein science evolved, that blame narrowed — and LDL became the primary target. Because LDL-derived cholesterol appears inside arterial plaque, it was assumed to be the cause of plaque.

Earlier chapters have already made the reality clear:

- LDL responds to arterial injury; it does not initiate it.
- LDL becomes dangerous only in a damaged metabolic environment.
- Diets high in sugar, refined carbs, and seed oils create that environment — not saturated fat.

Keys' framework turned LDL into the centerpiece of cardiology for decades. Even today, many clinics still operate within that outdated model.

Japan and France weren't anomalies — they were warnings. They showed that saturated fat alone could not predict heart disease, and that metabolic health mattered far more than any single nutrient.

But nuance doesn't win against a slogan. And Keys' slogan became policy.

The Legacy of a Convenient Error

Eisenhower's heart attack set the stage. Keys supplied the narrative. Institutions gave it authority. Food companies monetized it.

The result was a low-fat, high-sugar, high–seed oil diet that reshaped human biology in a single generation.

Keys wasn't malicious. But his theory — amplified by cultural momentum and corporate incentives — became the spark for half a century of misguided dietary policy.

The consequences are still unfolding: rising metabolic disease, obesity, diabetes, fatty-liver disease, and chronic inflammation.

Not because people eat fat — but because we've been told not to.

Where the Story Goes Next

Keys explained how the war on fat began.

The next chapter explains why losing that war was inevitable:

And it's where the real metabolic disaster began.

CHAPTER 11

The Fat Switch: When Industry Replaced Nature

For nearly two million years, humans evolved on a diet rich in natural fat. Fat wasn't optional — it was the fuel that made us human.

The human brain is one of the most energy-hungry organs on the planet. To build it, nature relied on dense, stable energy from fatty meat, marrow, and organs. Without those fats — especially saturated and monounsaturated fats — the dramatic expansion of the human brain simply doesn't happen. Our endurance, our long-distance hunting ability, our survival through harsh winters, our capacity to store and mobilize energy — all of it depended on fat.

Remove animal fat from the evolutionary story, and the human species collapses.

Which makes the last century one of the strangest detours in nutritional history: the modern world became terrified of the very nutrient that built us.

For thousands of years, every culture cooked with the same simple fats — butter, tallow, lard, olive oil, coconut oil, ghee. You could churn them, render them, press them, or skim them. They were recognizable, stable, and woven into human life across continents and eras.

Then, in a single generation, everything flipped.

Natural fats were pushed aside and replaced by something entirely new: industrial seed oils.

The most radical dietary shift in human history didn't begin with nutrition science.

It began with soap.

From Soap Makers to Food Giants

In the early 1900s, Procter & Gamble wasn't a food company. It made soap — and soap requires fat. But animal fat was expensive and supplies of it were unreliable, so the company looked for a cheaper alternative. It found one in cottonseed oil, a waste product used for machine lubrication, paint, and lamp fuel. It smelled rancid, tasted worse, and spoiled quickly — but it was dirt cheap.

P&G hired German chemist E.C. Kayser to solve a simple problem: Could this industrial by-product be transformed into something usable?

Kayser's solution — hydrogenation — turned unstable cottonseed oil into a solid, lard-like fat that stayed fresh seemingly forever.

Suddenly P&G had a product intended for soap.

It ended up being marketed as food.

In 1911, Crisco was launched — the first major industrial shortening. Its origin wasn't culinary. It was industrial chemistry repurposed for the kitchen.

How Crisco Became a "Health Food"

Crisco didn't taste like butter, and it didn't behave like tallow. So P&G didn't sell it on tradition — they sold it on progress.

They distributed cookbooks, hired early influencers, sponsored home-economics programs, and filled magazines with ads promising a "clean," "pure," modern alternative to old-fashioned animal fats.

The pitch worked.

By the 1930s, Crisco was common.

By the 1950s, it was iconic.

By the 1960s, industrial–seed oils had colonized the American kitchen.

None of this was based on health.

It was based on marketing.

The Turning Point That Changed Public Health Forever

In 1948, Procter & Gamble provided the American Heart Association with a major infusion of funding — a $1.7 million contribution (roughly $22 million in today's dollars) through the sponsorship of a national radio contest associated with the organization.

That donation wasn't an act of charity. It was part of a strategy. Crisco, and the growing family of seed-oil products behind it, needed medical legitimacy. At the time, the AHA was small, underfunded, and largely unknown. By funding the organization, P&G gained something priceless: a national medical authority whose messaging aligned perfectly with the shift from traditional animal fats to industrial seed oils. The AHA gained money, staff, and influence. P&G gained credibility and market dominance. And the public absorbed the message — not because the science demanded it, but because the incentives did.

That single donation transformed the AHA from a struggling volunteer group into the national voice of heart health; gave it a publicity machine it had never had; and aligned it — financially and ideologically — with the seed-oil industry.

From that moment forward, the AHA needed a simple, marketable message the entire country could adopt:

"Saturated fat is the enemy. Industrial oils are the heart-healthy replacement."

It was the perfect alignment of money, messaging, and corporate power.

America's dietary compass didn't shift because of evidence.

It shifted because of incentives.

This is the origin story of the fat switch.

How Seed Oils Took Over the Food Supply

Once cottonseed oil proved profitable, the industry expanded into soybean, corn, canola, sunflower, safflower, and grapeseed oils. The reason wasn't health — it was economics.

These oils were:

- cheap to grow
- cheap to extract
- cheap to transport
- stable on shelves
- ideal for ultra-processed foods.

Natural fats couldn't compete. Butter spoils. Tallow congeals. Olive oil solidifies in the fridge. Seed oils appeared indestructible — perfect for factories and fast-food giants.

One turning point came in 1990, when McDonald's switched from beef tallow to vegetable oil. Every major chain followed. Then schools, hospitals, restaurants, and institutional cafeterias.

Within a decade, seed oils were everywhere.

Today, over 90 percent of supermarket products contain them.

Foods advertised as "made with olive oil" often contain a token splash in a base of canola or soybean oil.

The industry didn't remove seed oils.

It disguised them.

Even baby formula — an infant's first food — is built on industrial seed oils. Not because they're biologically necessary, but because they're cheap and stable.

The subheading here is something of a misnomer. Seed oils — at least in the concentrated quantities lining grocery shelves — aren't really food at all. If most people understood how these oils are made — extracted using petroleum-based solvents like hexane, then refined, bleached, deodorized, and reheated to remove rancid odors — they'd never confuse the end result with "food." That uniform golden color, identical across bottles regardless of the seed, isn't a sign of purity. It's a sign of heavy processing.

The Chemistry Problem Nobody Mentioned

Traditional fats are chemically stable. Industrial seed oils are not. Butter, ghee, tallow, and olive oil are primarily made up of saturated and monounsaturated fats — molecular structures that resist oxidation and remain stable under heat. They tolerate light, air, and fire.

Polyunsaturated fats are different. Omega-6 and omega-3 fatty acids do occur in nature, and in small amounts, they have always been part of the human diet. They're found in nuts, seeds, eggs, and animal fat — diluted, balanced, and packaged within whole foods.

The issue isn't their existence. It's their concentration.

To obtain the omega-6 load found in a single tablespoon of industrial seed oil, you would need to consume an unrealistically large quantity of whole foods — cups of seeds, pounds over the course of a day — something no traditional culture ever did routinely.

Industrial processing removed those natural limits. Servings of seed oils deliver massive doses of omega-6 fatty acids. The result is a metabolic environment humans have never encountered. In the modern Western diet, the ratio of omega-6 to omega-3 fats now approaches 15–20:1. Historically, that ratio was far closer to 1:1 to 2:1.

This imbalance matters because omega-6–rich polyunsaturated fats are structurally fragile. Their multiple double bonds oxidize easily when exposed to oxygen, heat — or even ordinary daylight.

And yet these same oils are routinely heated past 400°F for hours at a time in commercial fryers.

If simple daylight exposure is enough to initiate oxidation, prolonged exposure to industrial heat doesn't merely degrade these oils — it transforms them.

The Half-Life Nobody Warned You About

Here's the fact that changes everything: The half-life of seed-oil PUFAs in human fat tissue is ~600 days.

If you stop consuming seed oils today, two years from now half the accumulated omega-6 PUFAs in your fat cells will still be there.

Two years after that, half of that half remains. And so on.

You don't "eat" seed oils — you accumulate them. These oxidizable fats become part of

- your cell membranes;
- your mitochondria;
- your inflammatory pathways;
- your LDL particles.

They destabilize lipoproteins, distort metabolic signaling, fuel inflammation, and make LDL more vulnerable to oxidation.

This is why LDL behaves differently today than it did in 1950.

LDL didn't change.

The chemistry inside us did.

Why This Message Struggles to Break Through

Every few years, someone with a platform tries to warn the public about industrial oils. The message spreads quickly — and then disappears.

Not because it's wrong.

Not because public interest fades.

But because the implications threaten enormous institutional structures: food manufacturing; agricultural subsidies; restaurant chains; pharmaceutical revenue; public-health guidelines.

It isn't conspiracy.

It's momentum — industrial, financial, and institutional momentum.

So the message resurfaces again and again, but never fully breaks through.

Europe's Partial Resistance

Europe held onto traditional fats longer.

Butter, cream, cheese, and olive oil remained central.

Industrial oils spread more slowly.

On a recent trip abroad, my daughter found a jar of Nutella with zero seed oil — same brand, same label. In North America, the first ingredient after sugar? Industrial seed oils.

Europe's food philosophy is simple: protect the consumer.

But even there, global supply chains are eroding the old boundaries.

Why This Chapter Matters

This isn't a chapter about cholesterol or LDL or plaque.

It's about the fat switch — the moment human biology and industrial chemistry collided, and natural fats were replaced by modern oils we were never designed to metabolize.

That shift reshaped: the food system; the metabolic environment; the way LDL behaves; the foundation of chronic disease.

To understand heart disease today, you must understand the world LDL now travels through.

The next chapter explains what changed in the broader food chain — and why institutions still fail to acknowledge the metabolic consequences of the switch that started with soap, marketing, and a single corporate donation.

CHAPTER 12

What Changed in the Food Chain

If you want to understand why cholesterol is wrongly blamed for heart disease, you have to stop looking at LDL itself and start looking at the world LDL was forced to operate in. LDL didn't change. Human biology didn't change. What changed — rapidly and violently — was the food environment.

Beginning in the mid-20th century, North America underwent the fastest dietary transformation in human history. In a single generation, people went from eating foods their great-grandparents would recognize to consuming formulations engineered in factories.

Once the food supply changed, LDL's behavior changed with it — not because LDL itself became harmful, but because the metabolic environment surrounding it became increasingly hostile.

And it all began with what replaced traditional fat.

A Quick Recap: The Rise of Industrial Oils

For nearly all of human existence, people cooked with fats that came from recognizable sources: butter, tallow, lard, olive oil, coconut oil, ghee. These were simple, stable fats humans adapted to over millennia.

Humans have long consumed foods like corn, sunflower seeds, and nuts — but always as whole foods, where the polyunsaturated fats were present in relatively small amounts.

What changed in the early 20th century was not the presence of these plants, but the use of their oils in foods; a single tablespoon of seed oil now delivers an omega-6 load that would otherwise require consuming pounds of whole seeds, something no traditional diet ever did routinely.

Cottonseed, soy, corn, canola, sunflower, safflower, grapeseed — oils once used for machinery, lamps, or soap were suddenly refined, bleached, deodorized, and promoted as "heart-healthy." Seed oils spread quietly through kitchens, restaurants, cafeterias, and eventually into nearly every packaged food in the grocery store.

The full origin story belongs to the previous chapter, but here's the point that matters for this one: replacing natural fats with industrial oils fundamentally changed the inflammatory and oxidative environment inside the human body. And that environment is the world LDL has to travel through.

But seed oils were only the first shock.

The Sugar Shock

Humans have used sugar for thousands of years, but it was always rare and expensive — a luxury, not a staple. European colonial sugar production made it more accessible, but it still remained a treat rather than a daily ingredient. The real shift came in the mid-20th century. After World War II, the

United States began producing vast surpluses of subsidized corn, and in 1957, high-fructose corn syrup (HFCS) was developed — cheap and potent, it was shelf-stable and easily added to processed foods. Within a generation, sugar was no longer an occasional treat. It was everywhere.

Unlike glucose, fructose is handled almost entirely by the liver. When intake skyrocketed, the liver buckled under the load. The result was a perfect storm: rising triglycerides, worsening insulin resistance, early fatty liver, and a constant drip of inflammation through the bloodstream — the exact conditions that damage artery walls and oxidize LDL.

HFCS didn't raise LDL levels.

It wrecked the environment LDL had to circulate through.

Sidebar: The Tobacco Playbook Didn't Die — It Moved Into the Food Chain

It wasn't enough that tobacco companies spent decades denying what eventually became undeniable: smoking causes disease — including heart disease. When regulation finally cornered them and cigarette profits collapsed, these companies didn't rethink their ethics. They repurposed their playbook.

They bought major food brands.

They hired the same chemists, marketers, and behavioral scientists.

And they applied the same strategy: engineer products people can't stop consuming.

Hyper-palatable snacks.

Bliss-point formulations.

Child-targeted marketing.

Shelf-stable "foods" designed to override satiety.

The goal was simple: replace declining tobacco revenue with rising processed-food revenue.

And the consequences were eerily familiar — ruined health, but in the case of the products of the multinational food, the result was skyrocketing obesity, soaring insulin resistance, and a food environment built to exploit human biology rather than nourish it.

Tobacco didn't disappear.

It simply moved from the lungs to the gut — and the health fallout has been just as devastating.

The Low-Fat Era — When Guidelines Broke the Food Chain

In the 1980s, North America officially declared saturated fat the enemy. Public-health agencies, armed with the diet-heart hypothesis, urged people to avoid butter, eggs, whole milk, and red meat. Manufacturers responded instantly. They stripped fat from foods and replaced it with sugar, starch, gums, stabilizers, HFCS, and industrial oils.

Supermarkets filled with fat-free yogurts, low-fat muffins, reduced-fat cookies, and "light" dressings. Consumers believed they were making smart, responsible choices. In reality, they were eating foods that spiked glucose, overloaded the liver, raised insulin, promoted inflammation, and created the exact metabolic storm that fuels plaque formation.

LDL biology never changed.

But it was now circulating through a body destroyed by policy and profit.

The Processed-Food Takeover

As industrial oils and low-fat products swept the market, a deeper shift took hold. Food stopped being food and became the product of formulations — mixtures of refined grains, sugars, seed oils, flavorings, emulsifiers, preservatives, and dyes designed for shelf life, consistency, and repeat consumption.

The change was subtle at first. A binder here. A preservative there. But by the 1990s, entire categories of traditional foods had been replaced by engineered equivalents. Today, roughly 60 percent of North Americans' calories come from ultra-processed products.

What makes them so metabolically disruptive isn't just the sugar or the oils — it's the constant chemical load the modern body must absorb. Emulsifiers alter the gut barrier and microbiome. Artificial dyes trigger oxidative stress and behavioral changes in children. Preservatives interact with liver enzymes. Pesticide residues from industrial agriculture enter the body daily. Refined grains digest so rapidly they behave like sugar.

Individually, each of these might be manageable. Together, they create a metabolic landscape our ancestors would not recognize — and one our biology was never designed to handle. Chronic inflammation rises. Insulin resistance spreads. Triglycerides climb. Gut health deteriorates. Visceral fat expands. And LDL, unchanged in its structure, becomes trapped, oxidized, or misread.

LDL did not cause this crisis.

It simply showed up in the middle of it.

Why This Belongs in a Book About Cholesterol

Because LDL has been blamed for the conditions created by the modern food chain. It is not a villain. It is a courier — responding to what your tissues demand and to the biochemical world you live in.

When the food supply shifted toward industrial oils, industrial sugars, industrial agriculture, and industrial processing, LDL began circulating through a damaged environment. That environment oxidized LDL, trapped LDL, and turned LDL into a symbol of fear — not because LDL changed, but because everything around it did.

Chronic disease didn't explode because people rediscovered butter or ate too many eggs. It exploded because we rebuilt the food chain around cheap inputs, long shelf lives, and hyper-palatable products that break human metabolism.

LDL didn't change.

The environment changed.

And now that you understand how the food chain reshaped the internal world LDL must navigate, you're ready for the next chapter — the war zone inside the modern human body, and what happens when LDL steps into it today.

CHAPTER 13

The War Zone Within You

You can blame cholesterol all you want. You can circle LDL in red ink, highlight it, underline it, slap a warning label on it. You can call it "bad" until the end of time.

But here's the uncomfortable truth: LDL didn't create the modern heart-disease crisis. Your metabolic environment did. And for the past forty years, that environment has been turning into a war zone.

This chapter isn't about LDL itself. It's about the battlefield LDL is forced to fight in. And that battlefield … is you.

The Human Body: Built to Adapt — Until We Broke It

For nearly two million years, humans adapted to almost everything the natural world threw at us. We endured snow and heat, famine and feast, migrations across continents. One generation lived on caribou and whale blubber; another on figs, grains, or olives. Biology flexed. We survived because we were metabolically resilient.

But our adaptability had limits.

We adapted to nature — not to laboratories.

What no human lineage ever encountered were synthetic sweeteners, artificial flavors, chemical dyes, industrial stabilizers, refined starches, and factory-engineered fats. For almost all of human history these substances weren't rare — they were unimaginable.

Then, in the late 20th century, the food supply changed faster than our biology could follow.

And the war began.

The Minefield We Now Call Dinner

By the 1990s, the contents of the average pantry no longer resembled anything our grandparents would have called food. A culture terrified of fat swapped butter for margarine, steak for cereal, and home-cooked meals for shrink-wrapped formulations assembled in manufacturing plants. Sugar became the default replacement for flavor, and subsidized corn turned into high-fructose corn syrup — cheap, potent, and everywhere.

Restaurants deep-fried everything in industrial seed oils. Supermarkets filled with brightly colored boxes containing forty-ingredient products engineered for shelf life, not metabolism. Three generations grew up eating foods designed for stability and profit, not nourishment.

This new dietary landscape didn't just challenge the body, it overwhelmed it.

Arteries inflamed.

Livers accumulated fat.

Insulin crept higher.

Sleep deteriorated.

Visceral fat expanded silently around organs.

LDL — doing the same job it always had — suddenly found itself navigating a metabolic terrain no previous human body had ever experienced.

The Silent Chemical Fire

LDL is not a criminal. It is a courier — carrying energy, fat-soluble vitamins, cholesterol for repair, and materials for cell membranes. In a healthy system, LDL cycles effortlessly, drops off its cargo, and returns for more.

But place that same particle into a body flooded with chronically elevated insulin, persistent glucose spikes, rising triglycerides, inflammatory cytokines, visceral fat, liver overload, poor sleep, and endothelial injury, and the biology shifts. The environment becomes corrosive. LDL becomes oxidized, trapped, or misread — not because it is harmful, but because the world around it is.

Plaque doesn't begin with LDL.

It begins with a damaged landscape.

LDL arrives only after the injury exists — and often gets blamed for stopping to help.

A Quick Return to The Fat Switch: The PUFA Time Bomb

Earlier, in "The Fat Switch," we saw how the rise of industrial seed oils changed the lipid makeup of human tissue. One fact bears repeating:

The half-life of stored omega-6 seed-oil fats is roughly 600 days.

Stop eating seed oils today, and years later, a large portion will still be embedded in your fat cells and cell membranes. These chemically fragile fats oxidize easily. That oxidation promotes inflammation, disrupts membrane signaling, and creates conditions that favor the production of smaller, denser LDL particles.

LDL didn't evolve into something new—but modern metabolic chemistry produces a very different LDL profile. That's the problem.

The Metabolic Explosion Almost No One Acknowledges

We now live in an environment where metabolic dysfunction is the rule, not the exception. Nine out of ten adults meet at least one criterion for metabolic syndrome. Nearly half have prediabetes or diabetes. Fatty liver disease — once confined to alcoholics — now affects children. Hypertension, sleep disruption, and abdominal obesity rise with every decade.

In a typical medical conversation, patients still hear doctors say, "Your LDL is a little high."

Almost no one says:

Your liver is overwhelmed.

Your insulin has been elevated for years.

Your metabolism is inflamed.

Your mitochondria are exhausted.

Your endothelium is under constant assault.

A complex metabolic collapse gets reduced to a single lab number.

Why Doctors Don't Break the Script

Most physicians aren't careless; they're constrained. Guidelines, insurance algorithms, board-exam doctrines, and liability structures all tell them to point to LDL as the central villain. Question the narrative and you risk being labeled fringe or non-compliant.

It is far safer to say, "Your LDL is high — here's a prescription," than to challenge seventy years of institutional dogma.

This isn't a failure of individual doctors. It is a failure of the system that trained them.

Where Heart Disease Really Starts

Heart disease doesn't start with LDL. It starts long before LDL enters the story — with chronic inflammation and oxidative stress; with years of elevated insulin and relentless glucose swings; with omega-6 dominance in cell membranes; with visceral fat accumulating silently around the organs; with fat trapped in the liver; with an endothelium battered by metabolic turbulence.

LDL is not the cause of the damage — it is altered by the damage.

Arteries don't clog because cholesterol is "stuffed" inside them. They clog because the internal environment degrades the very particles designed to repair them.

We didn't get sicker because LDL changed. We got sicker because everything else did.

Pulling the Curtain Back

If you want to truly prevent heart disease, the core principle is simple: Cholesterol is not the enemy. The metabolic environment is.

Once the food supply changed, LDL found itself operating in a fundamentally different metabolic environment. LDL didn't change but its interactions with the body did because the system it moved through did.

This truth has been buried under decades of politics, marketing, convenience, and institutional inertia.

But once you see it, the entire cholesterol story becomes clearer — and far more hopeful.

CHAPTER 14

The Modern Explosion of Heart Disease

Heart disease was not always common. In fact, for most of recorded medical history, heart attacks — the specific event we now recognize as a coronary artery blockage — were so rare that early 20th-century physicians treated them like medical anomalies.

There's an old story from teaching hospitals in the 1920s and 30s: when someone arrived with crushing chest pain, interns and residents were summoned from every floor. They rushed to the bedside because a confirmed heart attack was the sort of thing you might witness once in training — if at all.

Heart failure existed. Valve disease existed. But sudden coronary artery occlusion was unusual enough to offer a once-in-a-career lesson.

Fast-forward a century. Heart disease is no longer a curiosity. It is the dominant cause of death in the Western world — the background rhythm of modern healthcare.

So what happened?

Most institutions still recite the 1960s script: saturated fat, cholesterol, red meat. But the historical arc tells a different story — one shaped not by a single molecule, but by profound changes in how long we live, how we work, and how quickly our environment shifted beneath us.

The Shift No One Predicted

In the early 1900s, infectious diseases ruled mortality statistics. Pneumonia, tuberculosis, influenza, and gastrointestinal infections filled hospitals and claimed lives. Heart disease existed — but it was overshadowed by infections that struck earlier in life and in staggering numbers.

As sanitation improved, vaccines expanded, and antibiotics arrived, deaths from infection plummeted. Lifespans lengthened. With infectious threats declining, chronic diseases that had always been present suddenly became visible.

By the 1920s, heart disease had become the nation's leading cause of death — even though heart attacks themselves remained relatively rare.

Then came the postwar era.

Smoking rates exploded, especially after World War II. By the 1960s, over 40 percent of adults were smoking daily. Airplanes, restaurants, offices — even doctors' clinics — had ashtrays. At the same time, urbanization accelerated, physical activity fell, stress and work patterns changed, and the early signs of metabolic dysfunction began appearing in the population.

By the early 1960s, something extraordinary happened: coronary heart-disease mortality reached its peak.

Heart attacks had become routine.

The Decline That Didn't Solve the Problem

Starting in the mid-1960s, age-adjusted heart-disease mortality began to fall — slowly at first, then unmistakably. The reasons are well understood:

Smoking declined, and heart-attack deaths fell with it.

The drop in smoking remains one of the most successful public-health interventions in history.

Acute cardiac care improved dramatically.

This is where medicine truly shined.

- Ambulances became faster and better equipped.
- Coronary care units (CCUs) were invented.
- Defibrillation moved into hospitals, then ambulances, then public spaces.
- Thrombolytics, angioplasty, stents, and bypass surgery became standard.
- "Door-to-balloon" time — once an afterthought — became a race against the clock.

These innovations saved people during a heart attack — individuals who would have died a decade earlier.

But here is the part that rarely gets mentioned:

Prevention did not improve.

We got better at pulling people back from the brink.

But we did not get better at stopping them from arriving there.

Chronic disease prevention stagnated.

Dietary guidelines misidentified the villains.

Metabolic dysfunction quietly grew.

And the upstream forces driving heart disease kept accelerating.

This is why, despite the drop in mortality: heart disease never left the #1 spot.

It remains there today.

You don't become the #1 killer for 80 consecutive years because medicine failed in the hospital.

You stay the #1 killer because medicine failed outside of it.

Why This Chapter Matters

The explosion of heart disease didn't happen because humans suddenly became biologically incompatible with saturated fat or dietary cholesterol. LDL didn't mutate. Human physiology didn't break.

What changed was the world around us — socially, medically, industrially, and metabolically. Heart attacks went from rare anomalies to routine emergencies. Mortality soared, then declined, but the disease never left the top of the charts.

And here is the part too often overlooked:

Even as heart disease became the leading cause of death, the institutions responsible for explaining it kept pointing in the wrong direction.

For decades, national heart associations doubled down on the same narrow model:

LDL bad.

Saturated fat worse.

Seed oils the solution.

Statins the answer.

That model shaped food policy, medical education, restaurant culture, grocery shelves, and the very vocabulary of heart health. It shaped what doctors were taught, what families believed, and what industries marketed.

But it never explained the explosion.

And it still doesn't.

To understand why generations of patients were given an incomplete picture — and why the old story persists even now — we need to look at the organizations that shaped public belief in the first place.

We need to look at what the major heart associations still get wrong — and why it matters more than ever.

CHAPTER 15

What the Heart Associations Still Get Wrong

For organizations tasked with protecting public health, you would expect the major heart associations — the American Heart Association (AHA), the Heart & Stroke Foundation of Canada, and the leading cardiology societies — to evolve when the evidence does.

When food changes.

When disease patterns shift.

When the science moves on.

But they haven't.

Instead, they remain anchored to a narrative built over 70 years ago — a narrative born in a world that looked nothing like the one we live in today.

And that narrative — cholesterol → LDL → heart disease — still shapes everything from medical training to food labels to the ten-minute conversations people have with their physicians.

The foundational assumptions are outdated. The metabolic landscape has changed beyond recognition.

But the institutions haven't changed with it.

Not even close.

The Incentive Problem No One Talks About

We've already traced the moment the AHA transformed from a small, almost irrelevant volunteer group into a national powerhouse: the 1948 Procter & Gamble donation that rescued the association and gave it the reach, staff, and credibility it had never previously enjoyed.

That donation didn't just change the bank account.

It changed the incentives.

The AHA suddenly needed a simple, marketable message — something that fit on a pamphlet, a cereal box, a fundraising letter, or a heart-healthy logo. Something corporations could sponsor. Something the public could memorize.

LDL was perfect.

Easy to measure.

Easy to explain.

Easy to blame.

And — most importantly — easy to "fix" with a pill.

Meanwhile, everything that truly drives metabolic collapse — seed oils, sugar, HFCS, insulin resistance, liver fat, inflammation — was messy, political, and potentially threatening to the same industries funding the associations.

So they embraced the cleanest story available: saturated fat raises cholesterol → cholesterol raises LDL → LDL causes heart disease.

Everything — and I mean everything — flowed from that single assumption.

Guidelines That Never Caught Up

By the time the first U.S. dietary guidelines were published in 1977, the food supply had already been transformed. Industrial oils were everywhere. Hydrogenated fats were everywhere. Sugar intake — increasingly in the form of HFCS — had skyrocketed.

Yet none of these ingredients made it into the conversation.

Instead, policymakers doubled down on the diet-heart hypothesis. They warned the public about butter, eggs, and red meat, encouraged higher intake of grains and industrial oils, and framed saturated fat as the primary driver of heart disease. An entire public-health framework was built around a premise that was never proven, never tested against modern dietary conditions, and never meaningfully revised as evidence evolved.

And once those guidelines calcified into lessons in textbooks and medical-school curricula, they became almost impossible to correct.

Institutions rarely admit foundational error — especially when that error shaped half a century of training, billions in industry alignment, and entire branches of government policy.

Doctors Still Trained in a 1970s' World

If you wonder why your doctor still talks as if it's 1975, consider this: Medical students receive about twenty hours of nutrition training. Not per year. Not per semester.

Twenty hours total.

Meanwhile, they receive thousands of hours of training in pharmacology. They are tested on drugs, not diets. On prescribing, not preventing. On managing numbers, not environments.

The system trains them to treat disease with prescriptions — not food.

To lower LDL — not ask why LDL becomes dangerous in the first place.

It is not the doctor's fault.

It is the curriculum's fault — a curriculum built on assumptions from the 1960s.

A New Breed of Doctor — Finally Looking Upstream

But something is shifting.

A new generation of physicians — functional-medicine doctors, metabolic specialists, prevention-focused cardiologists — is rejecting the LDL-centric worldview entirely. They're asking different questions. Better questions.

If arteries are inflamed, why?

If blood pressure is high, why?

If plaque is forming, what upstream dysfunction created the conditions for it?

Instead of suppressing symptoms, they assess the system.

They examine insulin levels, liver fat, inflammation, endothelial function, triglycerides, sleep, stress, nutrition, visceral fat, and lifestyle — the real drivers of cardiovascular disease.

And when they address those root causes, patients improve.

But these clinicians remain a minority. The institutions haven't caught up, and most practitioners still follow a script written when hospitals sold cigarettes in the lobby and margarine was marketed as a miracle health food.

A Pill for a Number — Not a Solution for a Disease

This is not an argument against medication. LDL-lowering drugs have a place — for the right patient, at the right time, with the right risk profile.

But they cannot fix the real engine powering the modern heart-disease epidemic: a broken metabolic environment.

A heart association can slap a health logo on a granola bar.

A guideline can recycle a 1977 doctrine.

A doctor can prescribe a pill in ten minutes.

But none of that will stop inflammation, reverse insulin resistance, normalize triglycerides, or clear liver fat.

No pill will undo oxidative damage from decades of seed-oil accumulation or repair a collapsing metabolic system.

Suppressing LDL without fixing metabolism is like painting over rust.

It changes the appearance — not the outcome.

What Needs to Change

If these organizations want to reduce heart disease, they need to stop blaming cholesterol and start addressing the metabolic drivers that actually cause arterial injury.

What's missing is honesty — about seed oils, about fructose and HFCS, about ultra-processed food, about the failure to teach nutrition, and about the narrow, outdated obsession with LDL. Until that honesty emerges, the burden rests with individuals.

Institutions move slowly. Guidelines even slower.

But metabolic damage does not wait.

And that is why this book exists.

Because until the institutions catch up, the truth has to come from somewhere else.

CHAPTER 16

Statins: Fixing the Number, Not the Disease

Statins are among the most recognizable drugs on the planet, and their story begins long before your doctor prints a prescription. In the late 1970s, researchers discovered that certain fungi could block one of the liver's key enzymes necessary for manufacturing cholesterol. If cholesterol was the villain behind clogged arteries, blocking its creation seemed like a medical breakthrough.

When the first statin arrived in the late 1980s, it was hailed as a revolution.

Today, nearly 40 million Americans take one — roughly one in three adults over forty.

And here's the part no one says out loud: Statins are one of the most profitable drug classes in human history — generating more than $20 billion every single year.

Pfizer's Lipitor alone has generated over $150 billion in revenue over its lifetime.

You don't need a conspiracy theory when you have numbers like that.

If a drug makes tens of billions annually, and people must take it every day, for life, the incentives are brutally simple:

- LDL targets drift lower.
- Borderline becomes "high."
- "High" becomes "very high risk."
- Millions more "qualify" for lifelong treatment.

That's the real meaning of incentive: turn a lab value into a diagnosis, and a diagnosis into a lifetime customer.

For the pharmaceutical industry, statins were a jackpot.

For the population, the story is far more complicated.

The Decline That Happened Before the Drug

Almost no one mentions the timing: the steepest drop in heart-disease mortality happened before statins existed.

Heart-attack deaths began falling in the late 1960s and continued through the 1970s and early 1980s — twenty years before statins became mainstream.

Why?

Smoking cessation.

In the 1940s and 50s, about 40–45 percent of adults smoked.

By the 1980s, that number had declined to approximately 25 percent.

Fewer smokers → fewer heart attacks.

But once statins hit the market — precisely when the food supply shifted to ultra-processed, seed-oil-based eating — the downward trend didn't accelerate.

It flattened.

Heart disease remains the #1 killer today.

The Logic That Looked Scientific — Until It Wasn't

Statins rose to prominence as a result of a chain of assumptions that appeared tidy and authoritative:

Saturated fat is dangerous.

Saturated fat raises cholesterol.

LDL particles are found inside plaque.

Therefore, cholesterol causes plaque.

Lowering cholesterol must prevent heart disease.

It all seemed to fit — gears in a machine.

But every step in that chain rested on an assumption that was incomplete or wrong.

Returning to First Principles

A reminder:

- Cholesterol is a single molecule, $C_{27}H_{46}O$, identical whether in your bloodstream, an egg yolk, or a dinosaur fossil.
- Your liver produces most of it because your survival depends on it.
- LDL and HDL are not cholesterol — they are transport vehicles.
- LDL delivers cholesterol and fat where they're needed.
- HDL brings surplus back.

Biology built this on purpose. Neither particle is malignant.

So how did one number on a lab slip become the bogeyman of modern medicine?

Because somewhere along the way, medicine replaced biology with a narrative.

Doctors saw cholesterol fragments inside plaque and assumed cholesterol caused plaque — not understanding the toxic metabolic environment that damages arteries in the first place.

The story was simplified for mass consumption: cholesterol clogs arteries → LDL is bad → statins lower LDL → statins prevent heart attacks.

Clean. Marketable. Incomplete.

The Perfect Pharmaceutical Storm

Statins emerged during one of the biggest shifts in human nutrition: the replacement of natural fats with industrial seed oils.

As saturated fat was demonized, seed-oil consumption exploded.

As seed oils exploded, inflammation and insulin resistance soared.

As inflammation and insulin resistance soared, incidents of arterial damage multiplied.

More arterial damage → more plaque → more statin prescriptions.

This is what a sick-care system looks like:

Replace real food with unstable industrial oils.

Watch metabolic dysfunction skyrocket.

Treat the dysfunction with lifelong drugs.

Celebrate success because a lab number dropped.

Repeat indefinitely.

What Statins Actually Do — and Don't Do

Statins absolutely lower LDL, often dramatically.

But they do not:

- lower insulin
- reduce visceral fat
- repair endothelial injury
- reverse fatty liver
- fix mitochondrial dysfunction
- stop seed-oil-driven oxidation
- cool systemic inflammation

Because they do not fix the environment where plaque forms, they often fix the number without fixing the biology.

It's like repainting a collapsing house and bragging that the color looks fantastic.

The Side Effects No One Talks About

For all the enthusiasm surrounding statins, there's a quieter story your pharmacist won't print on the label: what happens when you interfere with one of the most fundamental biochemical pathways in the human body.

When you throttle cholesterol production in the liver, you don't just lower LDL. You disrupt a process every cell relies on — especially muscle cells and brain cells. And that disruption shows up in ways the glossy advertisements never mention.

Many patients experience the familiar triad: muscle pain, weakness, and fatigue. These aren't rare. They're common enough that doctors now casually recommend CoQ10 supplements — not because CoQ10 is some miracle nutrient, but because statins deplete it. CoQ10 is critical for mitochondrial energy production, so when it drops, muscles protest. The fix for the side effect is a supplement to patch the problem the original drug created. There is no universe where that qualifies as elegant biology.

And then there's what happens to the brain — the side effect no one wants to talk about. For years, patients have reported memory lapses, word-finding problems, slowed thinking, and a fog they couldn't quite describe. Some didn't connect the dots until they stopped the statin and their clarity returned. These aren't internet anecdotes. The FDA added a cognitive-warning label in 2012 because the reports were so consistent. The explanation is simple: the brain is composed of cholesterol-dense tissue. Neurons need cholesterol for synapses, for signaling, for membrane structure. Limit production too aggressively, and some brains push back.

Statins don't cause dementia, but they can unmask cognitive fragility — nudging a vulnerable brain into dysfunction. Families become convinced that "age must finally be catching up" to their loved one. Too often, it isn't age. It's the pill.

These effects don't happen to everyone. But they happen to enough people that pretending statins are risk-free is its own kind of misinformation — the kind wrapped in authority and given a final sign-off by a doctor's signature on a prescription pad.

The LDL Paradox No One Wants to Confront

Half of all heart-attack victims have normal LDL.

This finding has been confirmed across huge population studies.

If LDL were the dominant cause of heart attacks, this would be impossible.

Meanwhile:

- Many metabolically healthy people have high LDL but low triglycerides, strong HDL, low inflammation, clean coronary calcium scans — and no elevated risk.
- Guidelines still tell doctors to prescribe statins anyway.

Why?

Because the system treats the number, not the context.

Where Statins Truly Help

Statins do have a meaningful role. They provide secondary prevention: after a heart attack; to those with proven plaque; and to those with a high coronary calcium score.

Statins help stabilize lesions, reduce inflammation, and thicken the fibrous cap so plaque is less likely to rupture.

That's their real benefit.

Outside that context, the effect is far less impressive than the advertising suggests.

A Clue From Europe

Countries with lower seed-oil consumption have better metabolic markers, less chronic inflammation, and lower statin usage.

Not because they are anti-pharma, but because the environment is healthier.

North America breaks the system with ultra-processed food, then medicates the consequences.

The Central Truth the Guidelines Miss

Lowering LDL does not automatically lower risk. Not if the metabolic environment is still toxic.

LDL is a transport particle.

Plaque is the disease. It forms only when the arterial environment is damaged.

Statins can be appropriate tools in the right scenario. In the wrong scenario, they are a distraction — a way to treat numbers instead of disease.

A healthcare system would ask why plaque forms.

A sick-care system lowers LDL and calls it progress.

The Truth Patients Deserve

Statins are not villains. They are not saviors. They are tools — sometimes necessary, often overused.

But unless we confront the metabolic dysfunction that creates plaque in the first place, we can prescribe statins forever and never touch the real issue.

Because LDL is not the fire.

Plaque is the fire.

Statins do not change what keeps lighting the match.

CHAPTER 17

The Action Plan: Rebuilding Metabolic Health

By this point, you've seen why statins are not villains, but also why they are not a cure-all. They have a role in secondary prevention, in stabilizing existing plaque, and in high-risk situations. What they do not do is fix the biological environment that allowed plaque to form in the first place. That responsibility belongs elsewhere.

If you've been told you have elevated risk, early plaque, a concerning CAC score, or "borderline" labs, the most important question is no longer how to lower LDL. It's how to repair the metabolic terrain your arteries live in.

Target Visceral Fat First

Visceral fat is not passive storage. It is hormonally active tissue that drives insulin resistance, inflammation, endothelial damage, and abnormal lipid behavior. In most cases, plaque formation occurs alongside this metabolic dysfunction, not because cholesterol mysteriously turned hostile.

Reducing visceral fat improves insulin sensitivity, lowers triglycerides, increases HDL function, and calms the inflammatory signals that damage arteries. No medication replaces this effect.

Move to Control Glucose, Not to Burn Calories

One of the most effective interventions requires no gym membership. Walking for 20 to 30 minutes after meals allows muscles to absorb glucose without relying on insulin. This flattens post-meal spikes, reduces fat delivery to the liver, and lowers triglyceride production.

This is not exercise in the traditional sense. It is glucose management.

When structured exercise is added, moderate, sustainable movement matters more than intensity. Zone-2 activity — where breathing is steady and conversation is possible — improves mitochondrial function, fat oxidation, and insulin sensitivity. Excessive high-intensity cardio in metabolically unhealthy individuals often backfires by increasing stress hormones and inflammation.

Eat to Calm the Metabolic Storm

Ultra-processed food disrupts metabolism regardless of calorie count. Industrial seed oils oxidize easily, embed in cell membranes, and promote inflammation. Removing them from the diet reduces metabolic stress at the cellular level.

Saturated fat does not cause heart disease in isolation. In a low-insulin environment, it improves satiety and stabilizes blood sugar. Healthy carbohydrates still matter, but quantity and quality are critical. For many insulin-resistant adults, keeping carbohydrates under roughly one hundred grams per day — prioritizing whole foods and fruit over refined starch — produces dramatic improvements in triglycerides, insulin, and visceral fat.

This is not deprivation. It is alignment.

Support Arterial Function, Don't Outsource Repair to Supplements

Certain nutrients support the biology of repair. Adequate vitamin D supports insulin sensitivity and inflammation control, but dosing should be guided by blood levels, not guesswork. Vitamin K2 helps direct calcium away from arteries and toward bone, particularly when vitamin D intake increases. Magnesium supports vascular tone, glucose regulation, and sleep quality. CoQ10 supports mitochondrial energy production, especially for those using statins.

Supplements assist recovery. They do not replace it.

Protect Sleep Like a Medical Intervention

Repair happens during sleep. Not just any sleep, but deep and REM sleep. For most adults, at least 60 minutes of deep sleep and adequate REM are required for metabolic regulation, hormonal balance, and vascular repair.

Poor sleep raises insulin, increases cortisol, worsens inflammation, and accelerates visceral fat accumulation. No dietary strategy can overcome chronically fragmented or shallow sleep.

Consistent sleep timing, morning-light exposure, evening darkness, nasal breathing, and stress reduction are not lifestyle hacks. They are foundational to cardiovascular health.

Breathe, Relax, and Restore Nitric Oxide

Chronic stress keeps the body in fight-or-flight mode, impairing blood-vessel function and nitric-oxide signaling. Slow nasal breathing and extended exhalation help shift the nervous system toward repair.

Certain whole foods — including leafy greens, beets, garlic, citrus, and pomegranate — support nitric-oxide production and endothelial health. These work best in a low-inflammation environment, not as stand-alone fixes.

The Bottom Line

Plaque does not form because your body failed to manage cholesterol. It forms because the metabolic environment became hostile. Statins can stabilize damage when necessary. Vitamins can support repair. But only improvements in metabolism change the terrain. The bottom line is: Fixing the environment treats the disease.

There are more advanced diagnostics and individualized interventions that can be useful in specific clinical situations, but exploring those in detail is beyond the scope of this guide. The goal here is not to replace medical care, but to restore context — to help you understand why plaque forms, why lowering LDL alone often falls short, and why repairing the metabolic environment matters more than chasing a single number.

CHAPTER 18

The Algorithm Doctor

If you want to understand why people are confused about heart disease, cholesterol, fat, seed oils, LDL, statins, and metabolic health, you don't need a medical journal.

Just open your phone.

In 5 minutes, an ordinary person looking for clarity gets hit with the nutritional equivalent of whiplash. One doctor swears saturated fat is killing you. A nutrition Ph.D. insists PUFAs are not only safe but "heart-protective." A metabolic researcher says seed oils drive inflammation. Another calls that claim "internet nonsense." One expert tells you LDL predicts your fate. Another argues LDL means nothing without context.

Same topic.

Same confidence.

Opposite universes.

It's no wonder people feel discouraged. Imagine earnestly trying to improve your health — maybe after a scary blood test — and within seconds, TikTok pitches you into a gladiator match of conflicting authorities. Advice that should feel empowering instead feels paralyzing.

A Clarification Before We Continue

This isn't a TikTok problem. The same spectacle plays out on YouTube, Instagram, Facebook, Twitter/X — anywhere complex science gets crushed into 15-second sound bites. TikTok just exposes the chaos in fast-forward.

The Performance of Authority

Watch long enough and a pattern appears. Many videos start with: "Hi, I'm Dr. _____, and I'm a board-certified cardiologist."

That's not an introduction.

It's a pre-emptive victory lap — an attempt to win the argument before it begins.

But credentials only prove someone passed exams at some point in the past. They don't guarantee an understanding of metabolism, an ability to interpret new evidence, or freedom from outdated guidelines.

Some trained when saturated fat was Public Enemy #1.

Some updated their thinking when seed oils took over the food supply.

Some study metabolic health deeply.

Some still speak as if it's 1993.

Social media places all of them on the same stage — and once they're there, something more powerful than training takes over: confidence.

Algorithms reward confidence, not accuracy.

Short videos reward swagger, not nuance.

Humans reward whoever sounds most certain — especially when fear is involved. Which creates the paradox: the people who know the most often speak carefully; the people who know the least often speak loudly.

Guess which ones go viral?

The "Confident Cardiologist" Problem

I recently watched a charismatic cardiologist — perfect lighting, perfect delivery — declare saturated fat deadly in one clip and seed oils perfectly safe in the next.

No discussion of lipid peroxidation.

No biochemistry.

No mention of omega-6 overload or modern metabolic dysfunction.

Just eyebrows, smirks, and dramatic sighs.

He wasn't winning the scientific argument.

He was winning the algorithm.

Why Social-Media Medicine Feels Like Chaos

First, people aren't talking about the same biology.

One doctor discusses LDL concentration.

Another, particle count.

Another, particle size.

Another, oxidation.

Another talks about LDL levels within the context of metabolic syndrome.

Another about LDL in marathon runners.

To viewers, it looks like disagreement. In reality, these are different contexts flattened into a single argument.

Second, everyone draws from different slices of the evidence — statin trials, Ornish studies, Virta data,

Framingham Offspring, pharmaceutical reviews, biohacker experiments. Most people never learn how to interpret a study; they only learn how to repeat a slogan.

Third, slogans spread faster than physiology:

"Tallow is poison!"

"Seed oils save lives!"

"Butter kills!"

"Canola cures heart disease!"

"Statins for everyone!"

"Statins for no one!"

These aren't arguments.

They're branding.

Fragments of complex biology are stripped of context, amplified by platforms that reward certainty over understanding.

The Real Lesson

Scroll long enough and certain truths becomes obvious:

Credentials don't guarantee truth.

Algorithms don't reward accuracy.

And people desperately searching for clarity end up more confused than when they started.

If you don't understand insulin resistance, inflammation, triglycerides, oxidation, endothelial injury, mitochondrial function, plaque biology, and metabolic context, you're left guessing.

And when experts contradict each other with equal certainty, guessing feels like failure.

The Point of This Chapter

This chapter isn't trying to recruit you into a medical tribe. It's giving you the lens to understand why the battlefield looks like chaos.

Some doctors understand metabolic health deeply.

Some cling to LDL-only models built in the 1960s.

Some are brilliant clinicians but mediocre communicators.

Some are brilliant communicators who barely understand lipid biology.

Some are experts; some simply play one online.

And platforms treat them all as interchangeable tiles on your For You feed.

The takeaway isn't cynicism. It's realism: online, confidence beats evidence every time. That's why the next chapter matters — because once you understand how research is funded, spun, interpreted, and weaponized, you'll understand why an algorithm should never hold a stethoscope to your heart.

CHAPTER 19

Two Paradigms

If you listen to two cardiologists discuss heart disease, you might swear they're practicing in different universes. One warns intensely about saturated fat, emphasizes the dangers of elevated LDL, and cites large clinical trials showing that statins save lives. The other talks almost entirely about insulin resistance, inflammation, triglycerides, liver fat, nitric oxide, mitochondrial dysfunction, and seed-oil oxidation—mentioning LDL only as a downstream marker in a much larger metabolic story.

Same degree.

Same license.

Same journals.

Completely different worldviews.

Unlike the social-media carnival—where "experts" include pharmacists, dietitians, chiropractors, fitness influencers, and biohackers with ring lights—these two camps are both legitimate cardiologists.

So how can equally trained specialists disagree so profoundly?

Because they were trained inside different paradigms.

The Traditional Paradigm

Born in the 1960s and crystallized by the 1990s, the traditional model is clean, linear, and comforting in its simplicity:

Saturated fat raises cholesterol → cholesterol raises LDL → LDL causes plaque → statins lower LDL → statins prevent heart attacks.

Its elegance made it irresistible. So did medical-school curricula, continuing-education requirements, pharmaceutical influence, and the inertia of institutional consensus.

In this worldview, LDL is the primary villain. Lowering it is the primary mission. Everything else is a side plot.

The Metabolic Paradigm

The newer model emerges from modern evidence in endocrinology, inflammation biology, mitochondrial science, lipid metabolism, and advanced imaging. Instead of examining LDL in isolation, it looks upstream—at:

- insulin resistance
- visceral fat
- oxidative stress
- chronic inflammation
- endothelial dysfunction
- liver overload
- glucose volatility
- mitochondrial impairment
- omega-6 accumulation in cell membranes

Traditional cardiology sees LDL as the fire.

Metabolic cardiology sees LDL as the fire truck arriving at an existing fire.

Patients caught between these factions often assume the traditional paradigm must be correct because it has history behind it—or that the metabolic paradigm must be correct because it better describes the chronic-disease landscape of modern life.

This chapter doesn't pretend both are equal.

It explains how the divide formed, and why the interpretations differ so dramatically.

Relative vs. Absolute Risk: The First Source of Confusion

Nearly every major statin trial reports benefits in relative terms rather than absolute ones.

If your risk drops from 2 in 100 to 1 in 100, the absolute improvement is one percentage point.

The relative improvement is 50 percent.

Guess which number appears in abstracts, lectures, guidelines, and advertisements.

Traditional cardiologists see the "50-percent reduction" and conclude statins offer major protection.

Metabolic cardiologists zoom out and ask: Does this meaningfully change a person's real-world risk or life expectancy?

For most people without measurable plaque, the honest answer is: not really.

Long-term statin benefit in primary prevention is often measured in days, not years.

Healthy-User Bias: The Invisible Confounder

Much of the evidence supporting low-fat diets, whole grains, and seed oils is observational. These studies don't measure metabolic health; they simply track behavior.

People who follow dietary guidelines tend to:

- exercise more
- smoke less
- visit doctors more
- have higher incomes
- avoid obvious health risks

So, when guidelines promote seed oils, the people who use them most are already the healthiest participants in the data set.

Metabolic cardiology argues that improved outcomes are driven by baseline metabolic health; seed oil consumption merely tags along as a correlated behavior not the cause.

Same dataset.

Opposite conclusion.

Only one paradigm acknowledges the hidden variables.

Industry Doesn't Need to Fake Results— Just Shape the Questions

Pharmaceutical influence rarely shows up as manipulated data. It shows up in study design.

If the goal is to make LDL reduction look like success, trials can be structured to:

- pick endpoints LDL is guaranteed to influence
- compare a new drug to a weak control
- exclude metabolically healthy people with high LDL

- run too briefly for harms to appear
- define success purely as LDL reduction

The data remain technically "honest," but the framework is biased from the start.

Traditional cardiology accepts these results at face value.

Metabolic cardiology asks: Why didn't they measure the upstream causes of plaque?

The LDL Assumption Baked Into Research

Here is the deepest flaw in half a century of lipid science: Most research assumes LDL causes heart disease before the study even begins.

That assumption shapes:

- participant selection
- statistical models
- outcome definitions
- interpretation of contradictions
- what gets dismissed as anomaly

If LDL rises in unhealthy people, LDL gets blamed.

If LDL rises in healthy people, those people are removed from the dataset.

If statins lower LDL but fail to improve inflammation or insulin resistance, the trial still declares success—because success was defined as lowering LDL.

Traditional cardiology sees this as sound science.

Metabolic cardiology sees circular reasoning wearing a lab coat.

No one is lying.

They're simply standing on different foundations.

The Missing Measurements

Most cardiovascular studies never measured the forces that actually initiate plaque:

- fasting insulin
- triglyceride patterns
- visceral fat
- liver fat
- omega-6 load
- oxidative stress
- endothelial function
- mitochondrial impairment

Athletes, sedentary adults, obese patients, insulin-resistant patients, and metabolically healthy individuals were routinely mixed into the same averages.

Traditional cardiology accepted those averages as objective truth.

Metabolic cardiology looked at them and thought: This is like studying elephants and cats together and calling it "mammal science."

The Findings Everyone Knows but Few Emphasize

If you read the papers—not the headlines — a consistent pattern emerges:

- Half of heart-attack victims have normal LDL.
- LDL predicts poorly when triglycerides are low and HDL high.
- High LDL with low triglycerides show some of the lowest cardiovascular risk ever recorded.

- Many people with high LDL but excellent metabolic health show clean coronary scans.
- Coronary calcium scoring routinely outperforms LDL in predicting disease.

Traditional cardiologists know all of this. It simply doesn't fit the framework they were trained in.

What the Total Evidence Actually Shows

Strip away the noise and the message is clear:

- LDL becomes dangerous only in a metabolically damaged environment.
- LDL is often harmless in a metabolically healthy one.
- Seed oils, refined carbs, inflammation, omega-6 load, and visceral fat create the environment where LDL becomes dangerous.
- Statins help people who already have plaque—mostly by stabilizing it.
- Statins offer minimal benefit for people without plaque.
- Guidelines remain outdated because they were built before metabolic health was understood.

Traditional cardiology focuses on LDL because that's how the field was constructed.

Metabolic cardiology focuses on the environment because that's where physiology points.

Both camps want to help patients.

Only one aligns with the biology of modern life.

A Duty Too Often Overlooked: Check for Plaque

Before prescribing a lifelong drug, a clinician should determine whether plaque actually exists. Statins do not prevent plaque from forming; they stabilize plaque that is already there. Yet many traditional cardiologists order no imaging at all. They infer plaque from LDL or age and prescribe accordingly. This is why so many patients mistakenly believe statins "remove plaque."

They don't.

They stabilize it.

Lowering LDL isn't wrong—but without confirming plaque, it isn't precision medicine. It's guideline-driven guesswork.

Why Lowering LDL Alone Rarely Changes Outcomes

Statins genuinely make unstable plaque less likely to rupture. For secondary prevention, this matters enormously. But for people with little or no plaque, lowering LDL does very little.

You can suppress a number indefinitely, but if the underlying metabolic environment remains toxic, the disease process marches on. This is why statin benefit in primary prevention has always been modest.

Final Thought

This chapter is about choosing a framework grounded in physiology, not institutional inertia. It explains why two well-trained cardiologists can look at the same evidence and reach such wildly different conclusions. Once you understand relative vs. absolute risk, healthy-user bias, trial design, missing measurements, and the LDL assumptions built into early research, the divide stops being mysterious. It becomes obvious:

LDL was never the story.

The metabolic environment always was.

CHAPTER TWENTY

Beyond the Standard Checkup

At some point, you'll sit in a doctor's office — maybe with your GP, maybe with a cardiologist — and they'll scan your bloodwork, pause, and say a line millions hear every year: "Your LDL is high. That's our main concern."

This moment matters.

Not because your doctor is wrong, and not because you need to launch into a lecture about triglycerides, insulin resistance, or lipoprotein particles. It matters because the conversation that follows determines whether you receive a complete understanding of your cardiovascular risk — or just the narrow version medicine has relied on for fifty years.

Why Doctors Say What They Say

Most physicians are thoughtful, dedicated professionals. But they were trained inside a framework that treats LDL as the centerpiece of heart disease.

Medical school teaches:

LDL goes up → risk goes up.

LDL goes down → risk goes down.

Board exams reinforce it.

Guidelines repeat it.

Continuing medical education echoes it.

Pharmaceutical marketing circles back to amplify it.

So when your doctor fixates on LDL, they're not ignoring the rest of your biology. They're following the rulebook they were handed.

Understanding that shifts the dynamic from confrontation to collaboration.

The Goal Isn't to Challenge — It's to Widen the Lens

You don't need to debate anything. You should simply introduce context the standard framework doesn't include — thoughtfully and without tension.

Ask questions like:

- "How do these results fit with the rest of my metabolic picture?"
- "Are there indicators showing whether LDL is behaving normally or under stress?"
- "Would imaging help determine whether plaque is actually present before making long-term decisions?"

These are not "gotcha" questions.

They're invitations — and good doctors respond well to them.

The Illusion of a "Complete" Checkup

A standard annual exam feels thorough because it looks thorough. You step on a scale. They measure your height — as if that number has changed since the day you stopped growing. A blood-pressure cuff tightens around your arm. A lab slip checks the usual suspects: LDL, HDL, total cholesterol.

Maybe there's a quick question about your diet — something vague like "Are you eating healthy?" — and that's the entire assessment.

But look closely and the gaps are enormous.

Your weight is measured, but not your waist circumference, even though visceral fat is one of the strongest predictors of cardiometabolic risk.

Your BMI is calculated, but no one distinguishes fat mass from lean mass.

Your cholesterol is measured, but no one checks fasting insulin, the earliest sign of metabolic trouble.

You get LDL and HDL, but no one evaluates the environment those particles are operating in — inflammation, liver function, triglycerides, oxidative stress, blood-sugar volatility, mitochondrial strain, or endothelial health.

And unless you push for it, no imaging is done. No CAC scan. No assessment of actual plaque — the very thing we're trying to prevent.

What we call a "checkup" is really a quick inventory of legacy markers — measurements developed in an era when metabolic disease was uncommon that are, therefore, blind to many of the problems we now face.

It's not that doctors are negligent.

They're following the script they were trained to follow — a script written long before seed oils, processed food, sugar overload, and chronic inflammation reshaped the biological terrain.

That's why your questions matter: they bring modern metabolic science into a room still operating on 1970s assumptions.

Introducing Imaging Without Creating Tension

Many patients assume plaque can be inferred from LDL alone.

It can't.

Moderate or high plaque burden is the only scenario where statins consistently improve outcomes — because statins stabilize existing plaque. They don't remove it. They don't prevent it from forming.

This is why a simple question is so effective.

"Before starting a lifelong medication, would it make sense to check whether plaque is present?"

You're not refusing treatment.

You're asking for precision.

If plaque exists, the conversation changes.

If it doesn't, the conversation changes differently.

Either way, you move from guessing to knowing.

The Silent Shift: Many Doctors Want This Conversation Too

A growing number of physicians — especially younger cardiologists — are frustrated by the limitations of the LDL-only model. They know:

- metabolic dysfunction drives plaque
- lifestyle often outperforms medication in early disease

- LDL behaves differently in healthy vs. unhealthy environments
- imaging transforms prevention

But many lack the time or institutional support to initiate that deeper conversation.

When a patient opens the door, many clinicians are relieved — even grateful.

How to Keep the Discussion Constructive

Certain phrases work beautifully because they avoid defensiveness and invite collaboration:

- "Help me understand how you're interpreting these numbers."
- "What additional information would give us the clearest picture of my risk?"
- "Is this medication addressing the cause, or the marker?"
- "How do we know whether plaque exists?"

These aren't challenges.

They're bridges.

What This Chapter Is Really About

No single number determines your fate.

No twelve-minute appointment can capture the complexity of cardiovascular biology.

And no doctor — no matter how skilled — can protect your heart without your engagement.

You don't need to memorize studies.

You don't need to argue with a white coat.

You don't need to become a biochemist.

You just need to guide the conversation toward the truth:
Heart disease isn't caused by one number.

It's caused by an environment — an environment that can be measured, understood, and changed.

The questions you ask shape the care you receive.

And the care you receive shapes the health you keep.

CHAPTER 22

It Was Never About Cholesterol

We began this guide by defining cholesterol properly — not as a villain, not as a mythic substance that clogs arteries, but as a molecule the body builds with exquisite precision because life depends on it. LDL and HDL are not "good" or "bad." They are couriers — transport systems, repair mechanisms. What determines danger is not the cargo, but the environment. When the metabolic landscape becomes inflamed, insulin-resistant, oxidized, or overwhelmed, LDL behaves differently. It becomes trapped in an injury it did not create.

That shift — from blaming the molecule to understanding the environment — unlocks everything that follows.

Modern medicine still struggles here. We keep searching for a pill to do work only metabolism can do. Statins can stabilize plaque that already exists, but they cannot correct the conditions that create plaque in the first place. GLP-1 drugs suppress appetite and induce weight loss, but they cannot re-build metabolic flexibility or restore mitochondrial function. The underlying physiology remains largely unchanged.

Meanwhile, ultra-processed food continues to push billions toward dysfunction. Sugar, refined starch, and seed-oil-laden foods hijack hunger signals, dopamine pathways, and insulin regulation. People do not choose metabolic disease — they drift into it. A rushed healthcare system responds with a prescription, not a map.

But there *is* a map.

There always was.

We simply weren't taught how to read it.

Cholesterol is not the driver of modern heart disease. It is a passenger responding to deeper forces. Once you understand what truly shapes metabolic health, the entire risk conversation changes. You stop fearing a number and start focusing on the conditions that determine whether plaque grows, stabilizes, or never forms at all.

And here is the liberating truth modern research now makes unmistakable: you have far more control than you were ever told.

Cholesterol did not decide your fate.

Guidelines did not define your future.

The real leverage lies in restoring the physiology that keeps arteries calm, insulin low, and metabolism resilient. Do that, and the heart is finally given what it needs to do what it was designed to do — keep you going, strongly and steadily, for a very long time.

I did not write this book as a doctor or credentialed expert. I wrote it as someone who spent years reading research most people never see, connecting dots many guidelines still ignore, and asking questions most patients never feel empowered to ask.

Everything in this book rests on established, peer-reviewed science — not contrarian hot takes. If you turn to the appendix, you'll find the studies that form its foundation: large-population data, metabolic trials, imaging research, lipid-particle analysis, and inflammatory pathways — the pieces that finally make the story coherent.

And if this guide does its job, it may be the best ten bucks you ever spent — not because it offers "tips," but because it gives back the one thing the modern medical system quietly took away: agency.

You have more influence over your biology than any pill.

You have more power over your metabolic trajectory than any guideline.

And you are fully capable of changing the direction of your health.

Some physicians will bristle at that message.

Some cardiologists may dismiss it.

And the pharmaceutical industry would much prefer you keep reading pamphlets instead.

But if this book convinces you — truly convinces you — that you are not a hostage to a number, a guideline, or a prescription pad, then it has done exactly what it was meant to do.

Your biology is not broken.

Your environment is.

Environments can change.

And now you know how.

The Evidence Behind the Arguments

This appendix summarizes the most important scientific findings behind the principles in this guide. It is not exhaustive, but it includes the pivotal evidence that helps separate long-held assumptions from what modern research actually demonstrates.

Across thousands of studies, one theme repeats: heart disease emerges from metabolic dysfunction, inflammation, and oxidative injury — not from cholesterol itself.

Below is the evidence base that makes this clear.

1. American Heart Journal (2009)

Across more than 130,000 heart-attack patients, *half had LDL levels below 100 mg/dL.*
Why it matters: LDL levels alone cannot predict cardio-vascular events.

2. Circulation (2015)

When triglycerides are low and HDL is high, LDL loses most of its predictive power.
Why it matters: Lipid patterns — not isolated numbers — determine risk.

3. Framingham Offspring Study (2002–2016)

Individuals with *high LDL but low triglycerides and high HDL* had some of the lowest cardiovascular risk observed.
Why it matters: Metabolic context matters more than LDL level.

4. Lean Mass Hyper-Responder Cohorts (2020–2024)

Among metabolically healthy individuals with very high LDL, coronary imaging showed *no accelerated plaque growth.*
Why it matters: LDL behaves differently in healthy vs. un-healthy environments.

5. Keto CTA Trial (2025 — Emerging, Unpublished Research)

A community-led CTA imaging project initiated by Dave Feldman examined plaque progression in keto-adapted individuals. Early, not-yet–peer-reviewed results discussed publicly indicate:

- Plaque progression correlates most strongly with existing plaque burden, not LDL level.
- ApoB did not independently predict progression in metabolically healthy, low-carb individuals.
- High LDL in low-inflammation contexts may behave differently than high LDL in Western-diet contexts.
- Metabolic health — not LDL alone — appears to drive arterial injury.

Why it matters: If future peer-reviewed studies confirm these early signals, the traditional LDL/ApoB model may require significant refinement.

Note: Findings remain preliminary and should be interpreted cautiously until formally published.

6. Libby et al., New England Journal of Medicine (1995–2020)

Defined atherosclerosis as a *chronic inflammatory disease.*
Why it matters: Inflammation — not LDL — initiates and drives plaque formation.

7. Ridker et al., CRP Studies (1997–2001)

High CRP with low LDL was more dangerous than low CRP with high LDL.

Why it matters: Inflammation outranks LDL as a predictor of risk.

8. CANTOS Trial, NEJM (2017)

Lowering inflammation reduced cardiovascular events *without lowering LDL*.

Why it matters: Proves inflammation is causal.

9. PROVE-IT TIMI 22 (2004)

Statin benefit correlated strongly with reductions in plaque inflammation.

Why it matters: Statins stabilize plaque — they don't fix the root cause.

10. CAC Scoring (Agatston et al., 1990s–present)

Coronary calcium score predicts heart-attack risk independently of cholesterol.

Why it matters: Imaging measures disease directly.

11. MESA Study (2000–2023)

CAC outperformed LDL, HDL, and total cholesterol as a predictor of events.

Why it matters: LDL is a weak surrogate marker.

12. CIMT Ultrasound Studies (2005–2024)

Detect early, soft plaque years before calcification appears.

Why it matters: A CAC score of 0 does not guarantee the absence of plaque — particularly in insulin-resistant individuals.

13. Lustig et al., JAMA & Nature (2012–2016)

Fructose drives liver fat and insulin resistance.

Why it matters: Metabolic injury begins long before cholesterol is involved.

14. Shulman et al., Yale (1999–2021)

Mapped insulin resistance at cellular and organ levels — particularly liver-fat–driven insulin resistance.

Why it matters: High insulin damages arteries and alters lipoprotein behavior long before glucose rises.

15. Krauss et al. (1980s–2020s)

Identified small, dense LDL as a product of insulin resistance.

Why it matters: "Bad LDL" is a symptom of metabolic dysfunction, not a cause.

16. Reaven, Stanford (1988–2013)

Identified metabolic syndrome and its central role in heart disease.

Why it matters: Insulin resistance is the trunk from which most chronic metabolic diseases branch.

17. Ramsden et al., BMJ & NIH (2013–2020)

Reanalysis of older dietary trials showed *higher mortality* when omega-6 seed oils replaced saturated fat.

Why it matters: The traditional "replace saturated fat with seed oils" advice is not harmless.

18. Lipoprotein Oxidation Studies (1990s–2010s)

LDL enriched with omega-6 oxidizes more readily.
Why it matters: Oxidized LDL — not LDL itself — becomes trapped in plaque.

19. Mitochondrial Stress Studies (UNC, NIH, Baylor)

High linoleic acid diets impaired mitochondrial function and increased inflammatory signaling.
Why it matters: Seed-oil overload disrupts metabolism at the cellular level.

20. Monteiro et al., NOVA Classification (2009–2020s)

UPF intake correlated with obesity, insulin resistance, fatty liver, CVD, and higher mortality.
Why it matters: Industrial food chemistry — not natural fat — drives modern chronic disease.

21. Hall et al., NIH Metabolic Ward Trial (2019)

Participants consumed ~500 extra calories/day on an ultra-processed diet *even when macros were matched*.
Why it matters: UPFs dysregulate appetite and metabolism independently of calories.

22. Mozaffarian et al., NEJM (2006–2014)

Industrial trans fats sharply increased cardiovascular events.
Why it matters: Shows how engineered fats distort human biology.

23. Secondary Prevention Meta-Analyses (Lancet 2015; JACC 2018)

Statins reduce second heart attacks in people with established plaque.

Why it matters: Statins help when plaque already exists — by stabilizing it.

24. Primary Prevention Trials (HOPE-3, ALLHAT-LLT)

Showed little or no mortality benefit in people without known heart disease.

Why it matters: Statins are not universally beneficial.

25. Cochrane Reviews (2013–2022)

Found modest absolute risk reduction; side effects underreported.

Why it matters: Statins improve lab numbers more than underlying biology.

26. UK Clinical Research Group (2022–2024)

Estimated life extension in primary-prevention patients at 4–12 days over 5–10 years.

Why it matters: Demonstrates the gap between relative and absolute benefit.

27. STEP Trials, NEJM (2021–2024)

GLP-1 agonists produce meaningful weight loss but limited metabolic repair.

Why it matters: They suppress appetite — they do not reverse insulin resistance unless paired with lifestyle change.

Closing
Note

Taken together, the studies summarized here span multiple domains — plaque imaging, lipid behavior, insulin resistance, inflammation, dietary intervention, pharmaceutical trials, and ultra-processed food exposure. Despite their differences in method and era, they converge on a remarkably consistent conclusion.

Cardiovascular disease does not arise from cholesterol in isolation. It emerges from a damaged metabolic environment — one characterized by chronic inflammation, oxidative stress, insulin resistance, and ongoing arterial injury. Within that environment, plaque forms, progresses, and ultimately becomes dangerous.

Across populations, imaging repeatedly outperforms cholesterol levels as a predictor of risk. Across metabolic states, LDL behaves differently depending on triglycerides, insulin signaling, and inflammatory load. Across drug trials, reducing inflammation stabilizes disease even when cholesterol remains unchanged. And across dietary studies, industrial food chemistry — not natural fat — tracks most closely with the rise of modern chronic disease.

Viewed collectively, this evidence suggests that LDL is best understood as one variable within a broader biological context, not as a stand-alone diagnosis. The science does not point toward a single number to be suppressed, but toward underlying physiology to be repaired.

This is the story the evidence actually tells.

Glossary

AHA (American Heart Association)
A major U.S. heart health organization that issues dietary and treatment guidelines. Highly influential — and not always quick to update its views.

ApoB (Apolipoprotein B-100)
A protein found on LDL, VLDL, and other atherogenic particles. Each ApoB equals one particle — making it a better measure of risk than cholesterol content alone.

Atherogenic
Describes substances, particles, or conditions that promote the formation of atherosclerosis — the buildup of unstable plaque inside artery walls that can lead to heart attacks and strokes.

Cholesterol
A vital molecule used to build hormones, cell membranes,

and bile acids. Cholesterol itself is not "good" or "bad" — but the particles that carry it are labeled that way.

CoQ10 (Coenzyme Q10)
A compound involved in mitochondrial energy production. Levels can drop with statin use, which is why some people supplement it.

Cytokines
Chemical messengers used by the immune system. Some promote inflammation, others reduce it. Chronically elevated cytokines are a sign of ongoing metabolic stress.

Endothelium
The thin, delicate lining of blood vessels. When healthy, it regulates blood flow and prevents plaque formation. When damaged, it becomes sticky and inflamed.

Ezetimibe
A cholesterol-lowering drug that reduces cholesterol absorption in the gut rather than blocking cholesterol production in the liver.

Fatty Liver (NAFLD)
A condition where excess fat accumulates in the liver, often driven by insulin resistance and excess sugar intake — not dietary fat.

Foam Cells
Immune cells (macrophages) that have absorbed oxidized LDL. They accumulate in arterial walls and contribute to plaque formation.

GLP-1 Agonist
A class of drugs that affects appetite, insulin signaling, and blood sugar regulation. Often prescribed for diabetes and weight loss.

Glucose Spike
A rapid rise in blood sugar after eating, usually caused by refined carbohydrates or sugars. Repeated glucose spikes strain insulin regulation, promote inflammation, and contribute to metabolic dysfunction.

HDL (High-Density Lipoprotein)
Often called "good cholesterol," but more accurately a part of the cholesterol-recycling system. High HDL levels don't necessarily indicate low risk.

Hexane
A petroleum-derived solvent commonly used in industrial food processing to extract oil from seeds. After extraction, hexane is removed during refining, but its use reflects how seed oils are manufactured as industrial products rather than traditional foods.

HFCS (High-Fructose Corn Syrup)
A cheap, concentrated sugar derived from corn. Widely added to processed foods and strongly linked to insulin resistance and fatty liver.

HPF (Hyper-Processed Foods)
Industrial foods engineered for shelf life and palatability, not nutrition. Typically high in refined carbs, seed oils, and additives.

Homocysteine
An amino acid. Elevated levels are linked to cardiovascular risk. Often reflects B-vitamin deficiencies or metabolic dysfunction.

IDL (Intermediate-Density Lipoprotein)
A transitional lipoprotein between VLDL and LDL. Less discussed, but still part of the atherogenic particle family.

Inflammation
The body's repair response. Acute inflammation heals. Chronic inflammation — driven by poor diet and metabolic dysfunction — damages tissues.

Insulin Resistance
A condition where cells stop responding properly to insulin, forcing the body to produce more. Central to metabolic syndrome and heart disease.

K2 (Vitamin K2)
A vitamin that helps direct calcium into bones and away from arteries, especially important when vitamin D intake is high.

LDL (Low-Density Lipoprotein)
A cholesterol-carrying particle. LDL itself isn't the villain — it becomes problematic in damaged, inflamed environments.

LDL-C
The amount of cholesterol inside LDL particles. A rough estimate that often misses the real risk.

Lp(a) (Lipoprotein-a)
A genetically determined LDL-like particle associated with higher cardiovascular risk, largely independent of lifestyle.

Macrophages
Immune cells that clean up debris and damaged particles. In arteries, they can ingest oxidized LDL and become foam cells.

Metabolic Syndrome
A cluster of metabolic abnormalities that occur together — including high insulin levels, elevated blood sugar, high triglycerides, low HDL, excess abdominal fat, and high blood pressure — that greatly increase the risk of heart disease, type 2 diabetes, and stroke.

Mitochondria
The cell's energy factories. When damaged by inflammation or oxidative stress, overall metabolic health declines.

Monounsaturated Fats (MUFA)
Stable fats found in olive oil and animal fat. Generally resistant to oxidation and well-tolerated by the body.

Niacin (Vitamin B3)
A vitamin that can affect lipid levels at high doses. Benefits are context-dependent and not risk-free.

Omega-3 Fatty Acids
Polyunsaturated fats found in fish, grass-fed animal products, and some plants. Tend to be anti-inflammatory when balanced.

Omega-6 Fatty Acids
Polyunsaturated fats found naturally in small amounts in whole foods — but massively concentrated in industrial seed oils.

Oxidation / Peroxidation
Chemical damage caused by oxygen reacting with unstable fats or particles. Oxidized LDL is far more harmful than native LDL.

PCSK9
A protein that regulates how long LDL particles stay in circulation. Blocking it lowers LDL particle counts.

Phospholipid
A fat molecule that forms cell membranes. Cholesterol and fats rely on phospholipids for transport and structure.

Plaque
A buildup of lipids, immune cells, and fibrous tissue inside artery walls. Plaque stability matters more than size alone.

PUFA (Polyunsaturated Fatty Acid)
Fats with multiple double bonds. Includes omega-3 and omega-6 fats. Naturally present in small amounts — problematic in excess.

Saturated Fat
A stable fat found in animal products and some tropical oils. Long demonized, but not inherently harmful in healthy metabolic contexts.

Seed Oils

Industrial oils made from seeds (soybean, corn, canola, sunflower, safflower, grapeseed, and cottonseed), typically high in omega-6 PUFAs and vulnerable to oxidation.

Soft Plaque

Inflamed, unstable plaque more likely to rupture and cause heart attacks.

Statins

Drugs that lower cholesterol production in the liver. Useful in specific contexts, but not a cure for metabolic disease.

TG (Triglycerides)

The main form of fat in the blood. Elevated levels often signal insulin resistance.

VLDL (Very-Low-Density Lipoprotein)

Particles that transport triglycerides from the liver. Often elevated in metabolic syndrome.

Vitamin D3

A hormone-like vitamin involved in immune regulation, insulin sensitivity, and bone health.

Zone-2 Cardio

A level of aerobic exercise performed at a steady, moderate intensity that allows you to still hold a conversation. Training in zone-2 improves mitochondrial function, fat metabolism, insulin sensitivity, and overall metabolic health.

OPEN
LETTERS

- The American Heart Association
- The Leadership of the Pharmaceutical Industry
- Deans, Curriculum Committees, and Faculty of Medical Education

American Heart Association
7272 Greenville Avenue
Dallas, TX 75231

Dear Members of the American Heart Association,

For nearly a century, your organization has played a defining role in shaping how physicians, patients, and the public understand heart disease. Your guidelines influence medical education, clinical practice, research funding, and public perception. With that influence comes an enormous responsibility, one that, respectfully, has not always been met with the clarity or scientific adaptability the public deserves.

The central message promoted for decades — dietary fat is inherently dangerous and that LDL cholesterol is the primary driver of heart disease — has proven to be incomplete at best and misleading at worst. While science has advanced dramatically, your public-facing guidance has not kept pace. LDL cholesterol continues to be framed as "bad," despite growing evidence that cardiovascular risk is far more closely tied to underlying metabolic dysfunction: insulin resistance, chronic inflammation, visceral fat accumulation, TG:HDL patterns, and ApoB particle concentration.

We now know that half of all heart-attack patients present with LDL levels considered "normal." We know that carbohydrate quality, seed oils, oxidative stress, and glycemic variability play central roles in the development of endothelial injury. We know that metabolic health — not the absolute concentration of cholesterol — determines whether lipoproteins become harmful. Yet public messaging still leans on simplified narratives that obscure these realities and leave patients with an incomplete understanding of their own health.

I recognize that updating decades of public advice is not easy, especially when legacy frameworks are deeply embedded in clinical culture and supported by large institutional ecosystems. However, continuing to promote reductive concepts of "good" and "bad" cholesterol perpetuates confusion and delays the shift toward more comprehensive, metabolic-based prevention — a shift that could meaningfully reduce cardiovascular disease in our communities.

My request is simple: revise the message. Bring the public guidance in line with modern evidence. Emphasize metabolic health, insulin sensitivity, and inflammatory markers as primary drivers of cardiovascular risk. Acknowledge where older paradigms no longer reflect the current scientific understanding. The public will appreciate honesty, and clinicians will benefit from clearer, more actionable frameworks.

You have the opportunity — and the authority — to course-correct the national conversation on heart disease. I urge you to lead that evolution with transparency, humility, and scientific courage.

Respectfully,
Joe Bloe

To the Leaders of the Pharmaceutical Industry,

For decades, you have been central to our approach to preventing and treating cardiovascular disease. Statins, in particular, represent one of the most commercially successful drug classes in medical history. They unquestionably have a place in modern medicine — especially for individuals with documented atherosclerotic disease or very high-risk metabolic profiles. They can reduce events in the right patients, and their discovery was not without merit.

But their current use reveals a deeper systemic problem: they are prescribed far more broadly than the science justifies, largely because the therapeutic target — lowering LDL cholesterol — became an unquestioned dogma rather than a nuanced clinical decision. As LDL thresholds have been repeatedly revised downward over the years, millions more patients became candidates for lifelong medication. This expansion has aligned far more closely with revenue growth than with improved population-level outcomes.

Underlying this is a truth that deserves frank acknowledgment: the dominant incentives in modern drug development still reward maximizing profit, not optimizing long-term metabolic health. Statins effectively lower LDL-C, but they do not selectively reduce the LDL particles most associated with risk — the small, dense, oxidized particles that arise in a metabolically unhealthy environment. They reduce LDL broadly, including large, buoyant LDL particles that pose minimal risk. The science makes this distinction clear; the guidelines and marketing rarely do.

Furthermore, it should not be controversial to state that any drug designed to throttle a vital biological function will inevitably create unintended consequences. Cholesterol synthesis is not an optional luxury of human physiology

— it is foundational. Most of the cholesterol in the body is produced endogenously, precisely because it is indispensable for hormone production, cell-membrane integrity, bile acids, nerve insulation, and tissue repair. When a medication dramatically reduces this synthesis, side effects are not anomalies; they are predictable outcomes of interfering with an essential pathway.

This is not an argument against statins — it is an argument against presenting them as the default solution for nearly everyone with an above-average LDL level. It is an argument for transparency, precision, and metabolic literacy. The future of cardiovascular prevention will not be built on suppressing numbers but on improving the biological environment in which lipoproteins operate.

My request is simple: acknowledge the limitations of LDL-centric thinking, support research that distinguishes between lipoprotein subclasses, and align your efforts with interventions that target the root causes of metabolic disease rather than just its biomarkers. There is room for profit in genuine progress — and far more room for public trust.

Respectfully,
Joe Bloe

To Deans, Curriculum Committees, and Faculty of Medical Education,

Medical schools have long been regarded as the custodians of scientific truth, entrusted with preparing future physicians to practice medicine responsibly in an evolving world. It is in that spirit of respect — and genuine concern — that I write to you. This guide was written for everyday Americans who want to understand cholesterol beyond slogans and sound bites. But what the public needs in plain language, medical students deserve in rigorous academic form.

Medical educators themselves often remind students of a humbling truth: Half of what you learn here will eventually be proven wrong — we just don't yet know which half. This is not a criticism of medicine; it is one of its greatest strengths. Progress depends on the willingness to revise assumptions as evidence accumulates. But that humility only works when curricula evolve alongside the science. In the case of cholesterol and metabolic health, the evidence that has emerged over the past two decades now challenges many of the models still being taught. If we accept that some portion of today's instruction will inevitably be revised, then cholesterol education — still rooted in decades-old frameworks — is among the clearest places to begin.

Much of current medical training continues to emphasize LDL cholesterol as a primary causal driver of cardiovascular disease, often framed in simplified terms that no longer reflect biological reality. Meanwhile, the roles of insulin resistance, chronic inflammation, TG:HDL patterns, visceral adiposity, oxidative stress, and lipoprotein particle biology receive far less attention than the evidence warrants. Physicians are trained to manage numbers efficiently, yet they too often do so without sufficient grounding in the systems that generate those numbers in the first place.

Nutrition education remains one of the most striking gaps. Despite the central role of such education in nearly every chronic disease physicians will encounter, most medical students receive only minimal formal training in human nutrition — in some cases fewer than twenty total hours. I would urge medical schools to dedicate at least one full course to nutrition, metabolic physiology, and dietary pattern analysis. The public's growing interest in functional medicine is not a rejection of conventional care, but a response to its limitations. Patients are seeking clinicians who understand prevention, metabolism, and whole-system health. Medical education should be leading this shift, not reacting to it from the margins.

I recognize that curricula cannot pivot on trends or popular movements. But the principles underlying metabolic health are not speculative. They are grounded in biochemistry, physiology, and epidemiology. What remains is the willingness to integrate them systematically into training, rather than treating them as peripheral or optional knowledge.

This guide was never intended to replace formal medical education. On the contrary, it exists precisely because such education has not yet fully incorporated modern metabolic science into a unified framework. I would welcome — and encourage — a physician-scientist or academic institution to produce a comprehensive, peer-reviewed textbook on cholesterol and metabolic health that reaches the same conclusions presented here. Such a work would carry the authority and structure needed to reshape curricula, guide policy, and restore coherence to cardiovascular education. Truth does not require credentials to be valid, but credentials help truth become standard practice.

My request is straightforward: update cholesterol education in line with modern evidence, expand nutrition training, introduce students to metabolic and functional medicine principles, and prepare future physicians to treat cardiovascular disease as the complex, multifactorial process it truly is. Patients deserve clinicians trained not merely to suppress biomarkers, but to understand — and restore — the biological environment from which disease arises.

Respectfully,
Joe Bloe

About the Author

Gary Charles has always been curious — not casually curious, but relentlessly so. The kind of kid who couldn't let a question go unanswered.

That instinct showed up early. During his year in Mrs. Aaron's fourth-grade class, he earned a certificate from something called The Look-It-Up Club. This was long before the internet or smartphones, back when finding an answer meant walking over to a shelf of encyclopedias and digging. The certificate recognized that he "knew how to use encyclopedias" and was an active member of the club. But what stayed with him was the motto:

"We never guess. We look it up!"

It didn't just make him a curious kid — it made him the kind who memorized odd facts simply because they were interesting. His father used to get a kick out of it. When Gary was nine, he would proudly stand in the living room explaining to his dad's buddies that laser was an acronym:

light amplification by stimulated emission of radiation.

Here was this small kid, talking like a robot, cracking up a room full of grown men.

That mix of curiosity, precision, and a touch of showmanship never went away. It's what fuels the Joe Bloe™ Guides — clear, engaging, no-nonsense booklets designed to make complicated topics understandable for everyone.

Gary is not a doctor, scientist, or academic, and he doesn't pretend to be one. He's a lifelong learner who believes ordinary people deserve explanations rooted in evidence, not jargon. He writes about subjects that genuinely fascinate him — whether that's cholesterol, Montreal's infrastructure, artificial intelligence, nuclear power, aviation, human evolution, Fender guitars, or anything else worth understanding.

Whatever the topic, his guiding principle remains the same:

Ask good questions.

Look up the answers.

Explain them simply.

The Joe Bloe™ Guides are his way of paying that curiosity forward — helping readers make sense of the world, one clear subject at a time.

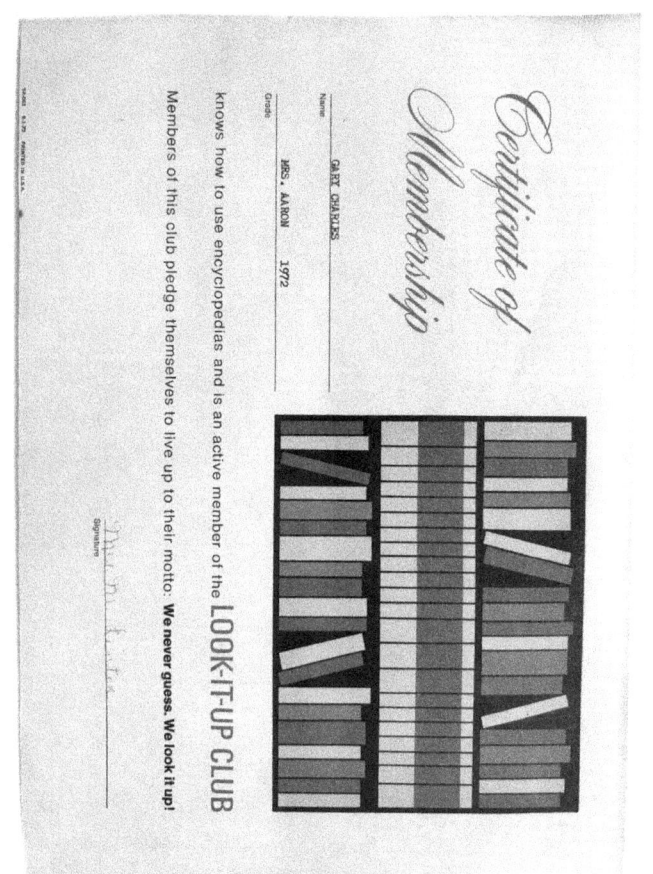

Certificate of
Membership

Name ___GARY CHARLES___

Grade ___MRS. AARON___   ___1972___

Members of this club pledge themselves to live up to their motto: **We never guess. We look it up!**

knows how to use encyclopedias and is an active member of the **LOOK-IT-UP CLUB**

Signature